The
MISLED ATHLETE

*Effective Nutritional and Training
Strategies Without The Need For Steroids,
Stimulants and Banned Substances*

CARL GERMANO, RD, CNS, CDN

iUniverse, Inc.
Bloomington

The Misled Athlete
Effective Nutritional and Training Strategies Without The Need
For Steroids, Stimulants and Banned Substances

The information, ideas, and suggestions in this book are not intended as a substitute
for professional medical advice. Before following any suggestions contained in this
book, you should consult your personal physician. Neither the author nor the publisher
shall be liable or responsible for any loss or damage allegedly arising as a consequence
of your use or application of any information or suggestions in this book.

iUniverse books may be ordered through booksellers or by contacting:

iUniverse
1663 Liberty Drive
Bloomington, IN 47403
www.iuniverse.com
1-800-Authors (1-800-288-4677)

Because of the dynamic nature of the Internet, any web addresses or links contained in
this book may have changed since publication and may no longer be valid. The views
expressed in this work are solely those of the author and do not necessarily reflect the
views of the publisher, and the publisher hereby disclaims any responsibility for them.

ISBN: 978-1-4502-9051-7 (sc)
ISBN: 978-1-4502-9053-1 (hc)
ISBN: 978-1-4502-9052-4 (e)

Printed in the United States of America

iUniverse rev. date: 5/9/2011

Dedication

To the two greatest athletes of all time – my son Grant and daughter Samantha – move over Nadal and Sharapova!

To all the men and women who serve in the US military – you are the true athletes and heroes of our nation.

Acknowledgements

This book could not be possible without the contribution of the following professionals who have provided their wisdom and expertise:

Donnell Boucher, CSCS

Donnell is in his fourth season as the Head Strength & Conditioning Coach for The Citadel Bulldogs, where he oversees the year round performance training for all of the school's intercollegiate sports. He is a Certified Strength & Conditioning Specialist by the NSCA and a Master's candidate in the Health, Exercise & Sport Science Graduate College at The Citadel. Boucher has served as a teaching assistant in The Citadel's Graduate Program, and has been published in American Football Monthly.

Rikki Keen, RD, LD, CSSD, CSCS

Rikki is a Registered Dietitian and Board Certified Specialist in Sports Dietetics and currently serves as the sports dietitian for Coach Tom Shaw, NFL Training facility at ESPN's Wide World of Sports. Rikki owns a private practice, Fuel & Fluids for Performance, LLC, providing nutrition services for athletes, BP wellness program and is a scientific advisor for FRS Healthy Energy. She also is an adjunct professor at University of Alaska-Anchorage teaching sports nutrition courses and conducting exercise testing in the UAA Human Performance Lab.

Michael Roberts, PhD

Dr. Roberts obtained his Masters degree in exercise physiology at Baylor and performed sports nutrition research in the Exercise and Sports Nutrition Laboratory. He earned his doctoral degree in exercise physiology at the University of Oklahoma where he continued to perform research studies in the areas of sports nutrition, exercise physiology, and exercise biochemistry. Dr. Roberts is currently a post-doctoral fellow at the University of Missouri-Columbia where he is studying molecular mechanisms that govern exercise-induced wellness. To date, Dr. Roberts has published nearly 30 scientific articles in peer-reviewed journals and has authored or co-authored five book chapters involving exercise and sports nutrition.

Beeta Little, BS, MBA, PMP

Beeta holds a BS in Human Nutrition and Foods and a MBA and Project Management Professional certification from the University of Houston. For the last two decades, Beeta has worked in the dietary supplement industry and is the current Sr. Director of Research & Development for Bluebonnet Nutrition.

Brian Appell

Brian holds a Bachelor of Science in Nutrition and has spent the last 15 years working in the natural products industry as an editor, writer and copywriter. He has collaborated on several books and magazine publications as well as worked in product research and development, formulation and education outreach. Brian is also a business advisor specializing in business and product branding.

William Arthur

Lastly, I would like to extend my sincere appreciation to my long time colleague, friend Bill Arthur for his editing, encouragement and words of wisdom – even though I never listen to him! A true marketing genius and consultant to numerous companies.

Contents

Foreword by Joe Theismann

Sports nutrition products in the United States have become somewhat of a "patch kit" for achieving muscular strength or optimizing performance. Unfortunately, one of the most grossly negligent sectors of the dietary supplement industry is in sports nutrition with products containing questionable ingredients, tainted products, unsubstantiated claims and misleading formulations. More and more athletes are searching for the next magic bullet to help provide them the edge in competition while placing training, diet and legitimate safe supplements second place. In addition, as the plague of steroid and banned substance use among athletes continues to spread in almost every sport (or at least those sports that are testing!!), the look to alternative natural nutritional support is being sought after and necessary.

The use of illegal banned substances continues to rear its ugly head in all facets of sports. Today, the National Collegiate Athletic Association, Major League Baseball, National Basketball Association, National Football League, National Hockey League and the International Olympic Committee have banned the use of steroids, stimulants and hormones by athletes due to their dangerous side effects. To me, the most important vehicle to inhibit the use of banned substances is through education. For this reason, it is with great pleasure that I write the foreword to The Misled Athlete by renowned nutritionist Carl Germano, RD, CNS, CDN and his team. As an athlete and football player, I was always told that I was too skinny, too slow, not tough enough, yet I never believed what people told me. I worked hard and long and rested well. Basically, I succeeded the old fashioned way and never was tempted to cheat the system by taking steroids or hormones. Throughout my playing career, I realized how athletes are susceptible to injury and that the human body was such a magnificent machine in its ability to heal itself. After my injury, I finally came to the realization that athletes were not infallible. Football is a very tough and physically demanding sport and I began to understand how damaging the sport can be to the human body. When Carl Germano discussed the concept of nutritionally treating the athlete as a patient, it all came together for me. He presents a concept, story and plan that have never been told before – one that is so critically relevant to athletes both young and old. By comparing the similarities and physiological consequences of the stress of exercise to that of a chronically ill patient, his case of the athlete as patient is clearly presented. His new mantra that if you help the athlete recover better from the stressor of exercise, you can optimize performance and help prevent injury is most intriguing and often neglected.

The Misled Athlete is both timely and important to athletes, coaches, parents and trainers as it provides the very needed education and sets the record straight as to what is truly important for the athletes well being. This book does it all by dealing with proper nutrition (diet and safe, sound supplements), effective training techniques without the need for steroids or stimulants and addresses the dangers of banned substances very well. To help stop the steroid abuse that exists, education about the hazards and side effects must be understood and the "other side of the story" is told in The Misled Athlete. The book will help all athletes understand that they can excel in sports without the need for banned substances and provides all the tools to help athletes recover and perform at their peak level – safely!

All of us in sports have an obligation to prevent athletes being misled. This is especially true of our easily influenced high school athletes who are vulnerable to the use of steroids and many of the worthless sports nutrition products in the market. Sound education as to proper training, diet and scientifically based supplements is essential early on. I hope that The Misled Athlete becomes required reading for all high school and collegiate athletes.

Joe Theismann

CHAPTER 1
Introduction – The Athlete As Patient

When my son asked my opinion about a sports supplement recommended to him on a popular internet forum, it was a question I had dreaded for some time and the impetus for writing this book. Knowing that he and all young athletes are the target of unscrupulous marketing about the next "hot" product to make them stronger, faster and bigger, I knew it was going to be difficult undoing the brainwashing and misinformation that goes with certain sports nutrition supplement companies. And I'm not alone in my concerns. The Food and Drug Administration and the United States Anti-Doping Association regularly monitor and find products being sold as a sports supplement to contain banned substances. A recent study tested 600 supplement products from around the world for substances that were not listed on the label and are banned by the National Collegiate Athletic Association and U.S. Olympic Committee. Twenty-eight percent of the supplements tested in the United States and fourteen percent of supplements tested outside the United States had banned substances in them with no disclosure on the label. This is quite unfortunate since the legitimate dietary supplement companies are overshadowed by the unscrupulous and deceptive ones.

Marketing hype, coupled with the intense pressure to excel by parents and coaches, has led to increased use of unproven or banned substances by novice and professional athletes alike. An informal survey by a former U.S. Olympic Committee physician showed that more than 50% of elite athletes would be willing to take an illegal substance if it would guarantee them a gold medal, even if they knew that taking the substance would be fatal in a year! While legitimate organizations and websites presenting accurate information about sports nutrition exist, they are also overshadowed by the marketing hype of unsubstantiated claims. The allure of gaining the competitive edge has led professional athletes, varsity teams, and even the weekend warrior, to experiment with everything from unproven nutritional strategies, such as excess protein consumption to the more deleterious anabolic steroids.

"More than 50% of elite athletes stated they would be willing to take an illegal substance if it would guarantee them a gold medal, even if they knew that taking the substance would be fatal in a year!"

There is a clear distinction between what is represented in muscle magazines and the reality of what the body can achieve naturally. That distinction is what this book attempts to convey. If you think that eating large amounts of protein, swallowing hormone analogs or, worse yet, experimenting with steroids is a sustainable approach to physical strength and performance then read this book very carefully as you have been grossly misled. It is my hope and intention that this book will help you view the athlete very differently than how you have done so in the past. My mantra is simple - if you recover better from the stress of exercise, you will perform better! An obvious, yet frequently overlooked concept. Optimal performance is only achievable if athletes are able to *recover* from the stress that exercise imposes on the body.

If you think that eating large amounts of protein, swallowing hormone analogs or, worse yet, experimenting with steroids is a sustainable approach to physical strength and performance then read this book very carefully as you have been grossly misled.

An in-depth review of the scientific concepts presented here may be found in texts and research studies for more detailed exploration. I have collected and tied it all together to outline a new view of the athlete. Numerous clinical studies have been published on the various hormonal, immune, and cardiovascular effects of strenuous activity on the human body. In many regards, those effects are similar to the same processes that occur during certain diseases such as in immuno-compromised conditions. Therefore, to address the multiple nutritional needs of the athlete, the athlete must be viewed as a patient. My clinical experience with oncology patients has taught me the apparent similarities between these two different "patient" populations. That is, muscle wasting, fatigue, oxidative stress, inflammation and immune suppression are common symptoms found in cancer patients as well as in athletes during prolonged strenuous activity (extended periods at 80% – 90% of your maximal heart rate) or in overtraining states. This book will cover the effects of exercise and how best to address them with diet, proper supplementation, and effective training techniques. In addition, the subject of banned substances and the dangers of steroids and precursor hormones will be addressed.

The Stress of Exercise

Intense exercise is one of the greatest sources of physical stress that athletes deliberately subject themselves to on a regular basis. Increased metabolism, heart rate, blood pressure, oxygen consumption, hormonal and even free-radical production are normal and transient responses of the body to physical stress. Remove the stress (i.e. exercise) and the body quickly shifts into recovery mode. Thus, the body adapts and becomes stronger. It is only during *recovery* that the body becomes stronger and capable of facing the next physical challenge. It is a thin line between proper training and overtraining that every competitive athlete walks and the consequences of hampered performance and injury that can result. Overtraining, a condition when the volume and intensity of an individual's exercise exceeds their capacity to recover quickly enough, and restrictive eating can exacerbate the physiological stress placed upon the athlete's body. Symptoms are physical (inflammation, reduced immune function, persistent fatigue, elevated heart rate, decreased muscular strength, tissue breakdown and weight loss), and psychological (irritability, loss of motivation and enthusiasm). Inflammatory markers and free radicals contribute further to muscle breakdown and impede recovery. Female athletes must take additional care to also avoid the "female athlete triad" (characterized by low bone density, amenorrhea and low caloric intake). Chapters two through five examine the physiological effects of exercise and the similarities between overtraining and disease states.

A focus on recovery is as important, if not more important, than the exercise itself and all too often athletes focus on the latter rather than the former. In addition to proper training, emphasizing good nutrition (with the right supplements) and adequate rest is the secret for the body to survive and thrive in spite of the rigors of exercise. Athletes generally recognize the important role nutrition plays in helping them recover and achieve their fitness goals. Depending on their sport, different levels of caloric intake and varying macro- and micronutrient levels need special consideration. The macronutrients (protein, fat, and carbohydrate) play a profound role in sports nutrition and the need for adequate levels of high-biological value protein to support muscular development and repair is necessary. The focus here is adequate high biological value sources not necessarily excess amounts of protein! Unfortunately, the marketplace has overemphasized protein and played "the numbers game," leading to the belief that excessive levels of protein intake are the answers to an athlete's nutritional needs. We need to go beyond excessive protein intake when discussing muscle maintenance and recovery. We must consider sufficient calories from carbohydrates and "good" fats as well. Finally, we need to examine certain nutritional supplements that can play an important and necessary part of an athlete's overall nutritional program.

Sports drinks, gels, caffeine-laden "energy" supplements and bars of varying caloric and nutrient content line the shelves of popular sports nutrition supplement stores in an effort to capitalize on the increased physical demands of athletes. The fact is that many of these products, especially energy drinks fortified with caffeine, only provide a false sense of energy and can actually impede recovery. They are not substitutes for proper nutrition and eating habits and should be viewed strictly as supplements to the diet. This book will review the pertinent diet modifications and sports oriented nutritional supplements that have legitimate application for performance and recovery. Chapters six and seven will specifically detail the proper dietary regimens that support the strength or endurance athlete.

Optimal performance is only achievable if athletes are able to recover from the stress that exercise places on the body. Diet, certain supplements, proper training, and rest are required. You have been misled to think that steroids, stimulants, prohormones, and excess protein are the answer – they are not!

In summary, the marketplace is littered with sports nutrition products claiming to be the panacea for increased muscle and performance. Additionally, the need to excel by professional and novice athletes alike has led to increased use and abuse of steroids with the hopes of achieving "greatness" at the expense of the body. There is no magic bullet and by focusing on the short-term gain that stimulants and steroids promise, popular sports nutrition products fail to address the multiple nutritional needs of the athlete. For reasons that will be outlined in this book, the biochemistry of exercise is very much like the biochemistry of chronic disease. Thus, the concept of the athlete as a patient acknowledges the need to address the critical issues facing the athlete (e.g., oxidative stress, inflammation, energy production, immune health, maintenance of lean muscle, etc.) through application of well-designed diet modification plans, effective nutritional supplements, and proper training techniques. *The Misled Athlete* focuses on these important issues and how to address them safely and effectively.

CHAPTER 2
The Exercise–Immune Connection
– A Dual Edged Sword

Frustrated by periods of listlessness and fatigue or suffering yet another bout of a cold or flu even though you are exercising? Isn't exercise supposed to be good for you and keep you healthy? Even though exercise is beneficial in so many ways, overtraining, not getting enough rest, or eating poorly can tip the scales and impact health for the worse. The immune system is susceptible to the stress of exercise, leading to an overtaxed or poor immune response. As we hinted to in chapter one, the stress of exercise is not too different than the immunological response to certain diseases. Yes, exercise! Every time the body undergoes strenuous activity, it reacts similarly as it would during certain illnesses. This chapter will show that every time an athlete leaves the field, court or gym, the response of the immune system is transiently suppressed and therefore requires support.

The immune system is one of the most biologically complex systems of the body. At its most basic level, its primary function is to guard against injury, infections or to facilitate healing. To do its job the immune system recruits an army of specialized cells with menacing names like natural killer cells and macrophages and

Leukocyte (white blood cell) differentials

Agranulocytes

Lymphocytes (23-28%)
- divided into T cells (kill infected cells), B cells (produce antibodies), and NK cells (kill infected cells)

Monocytes (3-8%)
- recruited to muscle during the acute post-exercise inflammation
- replinish macrophages and produce cytokines in muscle after exercise

Granulocytes

Neutrophils (60-70%)
- recruited to muscle during the acute post-exercise inflammation

Eosinophils (~2-5%)
- protect against parasites
- elevated during allergic reactions

Basophils(~1%)
- protect against parasites
- elevated during allergic reactions

lymphocytes like T cells and B cells. Together, they roam the body with total devotion to protect. The immune system also communicates with almost every other cell in the body, including nerve and muscle cells. This total integration allows the body to monitor our health and react quickly when trouble arises. Various chemical messengers called cytokines orchestrate this enormous task appointed to the immune system. Cytokines are to the immune system as neurotransmitters are to the brain. Just as the brain relies on neurotransmitters to exchange information to the rest of the body, cytokines relay information to and from the immune system. They transmit information from cell to cell, either stimulating or calming immune activity and inflammation (an important part of the immune response). This is an important point to stress: cytokines function to balance immune activity – telling immune cells when to fight and when *not* to fight.

Cytokines can be grouped into two broad categories: those that can cause inflammation and those that reduce inflammation. They control how long, how fast, and in what part of the body the immune system conducts its business. The myriad of cytokines produced during and after an immune response exemplifies the need for the body to react quickly to infection or injury and shut down efficiently when the threat has passed. It was originally thought that cytokine production was produced solely by immune cells. Recent evidence shows that cytokines are also produce by muscle cells and significantly increased during intense exercise. This makes sense considering how exercise affects the body. Strenuous exercise traumatizes muscle tissue that triggers cytokines to mobilize the immune system. Unfortunately, some of those cytokines trigger an inflammatory response. During intense or extended training (i.e. overtraining) prolonged exposure to inflammatory cytokines can have negative effects including muscle damage. In addition to an increased inflammatory response, various studies have demonstrated immune suppression after high-intensity training. Specifically, studies have shown that after strenuous activity there is a decrease in the concentration of protective proteins called immunoglobulins in the nasal cavity indicating that exercise impedes the ability of the upper respiratory tract to clear viruses and bacteria. There are many case studies and reviews by coaches and practitioners who report significantly reduced athletic performance during recent bouts of sickness known in some circles as "post-viral fatigue syndrome."

So, intense exercise paradoxically increases the inflammatory response while suppressing immune function, which leads to poor recovery and increased risk of infection (i.e. upper respiratory tract infections best demonstrated by the popular "J" curve below). This is apparent in even well trained athletes. Poor diet, inadequate rest, overtraining or poor training techniques exacerbate this effect while a balanced regimen of exercise, healthy diet and adequate rest leads to better performance, improved muscle mass and enhanced immune function.

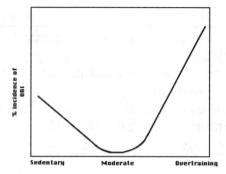

How Much of a Concern for the Athlete?
First, the Good News!

We know that regular, moderate exercise is very beneficial and can improve immune response and health. Moderate exercise reduces the risk of colds, flu, upper respiratory and other viral infections compared to those who do not exercise. Moderate exercise protects against inflammation, which is important for athletes to prevent injury and reduce the breakdown of muscle after activity. The key words here are "moderate exercise." It is an unfortunate fact that young athletes as well as professional sports players are pushed to the edge to compete and moderate exercise has no place in their training. Even for bodybuilders, the enormous amount of pre-workout stimulant products that push the body to do more work has made the term moderate exercise obsolete.

Now, the Bad News!

Research points to strenuous activity mimicking the pattern of hormonal and immunological responses we see in post surgical and immune-compromised patients such as those suffering from cancer. Several studies indicate that strenuous exercise produces an immediate immune response similar to the response seen during infections and trauma. We now understand and have identified several immune cytokines that are increased in response to exercise the same way we see them elevated in response to infections, tissue injury, or certain degenerative or immune-compromised diseases. Certain cytokines are destructive inflammatory ones and include interleukin-1 (IL-1), C-reactive

7

protein, tumor necrosis factor, and interleukin-6 (IL-6). Interestingly, IL-6 is considered both inflammatory and sometimes anti-inflammatory, depending on the nutritional state of an athlete and their ability to quickly recover after strenuous activity.

° **Strenuous bouts of exercise are associated with depressed immune function**

° **The chronic stress of heavy training can result in transient immuno-suppression**

° **After intense exercise, athletes go through a period of impaired immune response making them more susceptible to viral infections**

In addition, elevated IL-6 incites another inflammatory marker called C-reactive protein or CRP, which is present in many diseases including certain cardiovascular disorders and cancer. Research has now confirmed that high intensity exercise significantly increases circulating levels of CRP. So, if you think you can perform well when you're sick, think again. While elevation of cytokines and inflammatory markers are normal and an adaptive immune response, it is essential to reduce their levels as quickly as possible since they can contribute to muscle breakdown, fatigue, and increased risk of infection.

In Come the Hormones!

Along with affecting the immune response, rigorous exercise elicits the help of the adrenal glands to deal with this stress. They release hormones, including epinephrine, cortisol, progesterone, estrogen, testosterone, and dehydroepi-androsterone (DHEA) to assist in balancing blood sugar for an even flow of energy throughout the day and managing energy output when under physical or mental pressure. Again, this is a normal response that quickly normalizes when the stress subsides. Under prolonged bouts of stress, the adrenal glands may be over-stimulated and unable to meet the demands of the body, con-tributing to chronic fatigue, body aches, nervousness, sleep disturbances and digestive problems. Along with its effect on immune function, intense

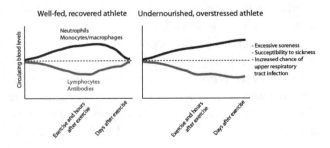

exercise taxes the adrenal glands, leading to increased cortisol production. The result is inhibited uptake of glucose into cells for energy production, suppressed collagen synthesis (an important protein for healthy joints), inhibited bone growth (via inhibition of osteoblast activity – the bone-building cells of the body), and protein synthesis (needed for muscle repair and growth). It's fair to say that you do not want elevated cortisol levels for long periods of time!!

Immune-Inflammation Connection – Burn Baby Burn!

The effect of increased inflammatory response resulting from overtraining is more than just the overt redness, pain, heat, and swelling seen in injury. Those menacing inflammatory molecules can reduce the function of joints as well as contribute to muscle breakdown. When chronically elevated, inflammatory cytokines dilate blood vessels in muscles and joints and increase swelling and cause pain. To combat inflammation associated with overtraining (as well as inflammation from other sources), nonsteroidal anti-inflammatory drugs (NSAIDs) are typically the first line of attack. Unfortunately, long-term use increases the risk of adverse effects such as gastrointestinal problems, ulcers, and kidney and liver damage. The other option is the use of anti-inflammatory steroids (different from anabolic steroids) to halt inflammation. While commonly prescribed steroids such as cortisone and prednisone do the job, chronic use actually has an opposite effect – they eventually impede the healing process by negatively affecting the production of collagen (important for your joints and tissue repair). Neither NSAIDs nor anti-inflammatory steroids are viable options for long-term use. For these reasons, a growing number of practitioners and laypersons alike are now seeking alternatives to reduce the symptoms of inflammation.

Do not rely on NSAIDs or steroids since chronic use can contribute to intestinal, kidney or liver problems. Long- term use can also interfere with your ability to heal damaged cartilage in joints.

Supporting Immunity & Reducing Inflammation Naturally

So, now that we know intense exercise transiently suppresses immune function, increases inflammation and certain hormones that can hinder the recovery process, what can be done to address this neglected issue? First, it is very important to practice proper training techniques to prevent overtraining. Working with and listening to your strength and conditioning coach is critical. In addition, immune support and muscle recovery require dietary manipulation (especially proper carbohydrate to protein ratio) and the use of safe supplements including certain amino acids and antioxidants, which will be discussed in detail. Proper immune function is a critical component for optimal performance since it is necessary to help prepare the body for the stress of exercise. Finally, adequate sleep, perhaps the most neglected component for recovery and immune health, is essential. Make sure to get eight or more hours every night.

It is equally important to emphasize that while dietary supplements are essential, they are only an adjunct to the diet. Athletes need to really focus on eating a well-balanced diet sufficient to meet their energy, carbohydrate, protein and micronutrient needs. While effective training methods and proper dietary manipulation is covered in other chapters, below is a cursory overview of dietary and nutritional supplement components that are helpful for strengthening the immune response and reducing inflammation. This subject alone can cover an entire book, so I have carefully chosen some of the most efficacious supplements to add to your nutritional arsenal.

Nutritional Support

You must understand that the diet and the foods you choose are the primary focus to keeping your immune system healthy. This is discussed more in chapter six but suffice to say modifications are needed to address adequate caloric intake as well as proper carbohydrate-to-protein ratio. While the use of certain supplements can provide benefit and support, carbohydrate supplementation is particularly important in preventing exercise-induced immune suppression. There is a strong connection between depleted stores of carbohydrates and fatigue, increased release of stress hormones, and reduced immune activity. In addition, incorporation of more alkaline, phytonutrient-rich fruits and vegetables are essential to a healthy immune system and reducing acidity in muscles. Therefore, the supplements listed below are in addition to a healthy diet – not a substitute!

Healthy Food Choices

- While simple sugars are important before, during and after strenuous activity, avoid all forms of empty calorie foods throughout the rest of the day (e.g., cakes, cookies, pies, pastries, doughnuts, soda, juice). Avoid carbohydrates with a high glycemic value/load (glycemic value/load, or glycemic index, is a measure of the effect of carbohydrates on blood sugar. The higher the value, the greater its effect on raising blood sugar).

- Eat plenty of alkaline foods such as green leafy vegetables, citrus and dark colored fruits (tart cherries, blueberries, pomegranate, etc) and nuts and seeds. The phytonutrients found in these foods contain proven antioxidant and anti-inflammatory properties.

- Incorporate more medicinal mushrooms into your diet. These include shiitake, maitake, king oyster and Portobello. Mushrooms are rich sources of polysaccharides (carbohydrate polymers) that help modulate immune response.

- Drink plenty of white and green tea.

- Eat healthy fats such as extra virgin olive oil (monounsaturated fats) and fish such as salmon, tuna, mackerel, and sardines, which are abundant in omega-3 fats. For you vegetarians and vegans, walnuts are also high in omega-3 fats. Avoid consuming excessive amounts of corn oil or other oils high in omega-6 fats. Absolutely avoid all trans fats (partially hydrogenated oils) still found in many packaged foods and fried foods.

Buyer Beware: If you see "0g" trans fats in the "Nutritional Facts" box on the label yet still see the words "partially hydrogenated oil/fat" in the "Other Ingredients" section, you have been misled to think there are no trans fats in the product. The label law allows a "0g" claim if the serving provides less than 1 gram of trans fat, but eating more than 1 serving of snack foods is commonplace.
Bottom line: if you see partially hydrogenated oil/fat listed in the "Other Ingredients" section, it has trans fats in it and should be avoided!

Supplements for Immune Support

Multivitamin/Mineral – One can make the case for almost all vitamins and minerals having a role to play for supporting a healthy immune system, but it is impossible within the scope of this book to cover such an enormous topic. While we would like to focus on having your diet supply all the important nutrients needed, the glaring truth is that most people do not eat healthy and several studies demonstrate that numerous deficiencies continue to exist. Since marginal deficiencies of many vitamins and minerals can have a negative effect on immune function, it is best to start with a good multivitamin that provides sufficient levels of antioxidants, B-vitamins and essential minerals. Additionally, since we do not eat one meal a day to cover our entire dietary needs, the "One-A-Day" multivitamin/mineral is equally insufficient when it comes to supplementation. Taking large amounts of nutrients all at once is not absorbed efficiently, ending up primarily in the urine! The best multivitamins are those that are taken two or three times daily. This way you supply key nutrients to the body over a larger span of time throughout the day. Also, the minerals should be "chelated" (a mineral bound to an organic compound, such as amino acids) for improved absorption and utilization.

Vitamin D – Because of its importance, this specific vitamin is highlighted in several places throughout the book. Over the past decade the research on vitamin D has elucidated its importance for immune health. Other than its classical role in bone health, vitamin D plays a crucial role in immune function and deficiencies can increase the risk of infections and illness. It is now known that all cells of the body have receptors for vitamin D and many cells of the immune system are dormant until they are activated by this nutrient. Vitamin D also inhibits pro-inflammatory messengers such as Il-1 and Il-12 that are involved in muscle breakdown. Unfortunately, we have been grossly misled to believe that the current Recommended Dietary Allowance of 400 IU (International Units) daily is sufficient. Scientific and medical communities are calling for increasing the daily allowance to several thousand IUs daily. Most multivitamin/mineral supplements will not have adequate amounts to satisfy most individuals. Therefore, additional vitamin D supplements are required to increase blood levels to support healthy immune and anti-inflammatory activity.
Effective Dose: 1,000 - 2,000 IU daily for several weeks and, if possible, request that your primary care physician measures your blood vitamin D levels. You will need to adjust the amount of vitamin D intake to achieve a healthy range of approximately 50 - 75 ng/mL.

Glutamine - Glutamine is one of the most abundant amino acids in the body and plays important functional roles ranging from antioxidant defense to supporting immune function. Immune cells such as lymphocytes and macrophages are particularly dependent on glutamine levels. Deficiency of this amino acid is seen in many conditions including cancer, inflammatory diseases, chronic stress, trauma, and prolonged strenuous exercise. During such conditions, blood glutamine concentrations decrease significantly and limit the amount available to meet the demands of the immune system. The results are poor immune response, loss of muscle mass and poor antioxidant defense. After intense exercise, depletion of glutamine can slow wound healing and muscle recovery. In addition, studies have now demonstrated the importance of glutamine in the adaptation and preservation of proper immune function during exercise. Lastly, the anabolic activity of glutamine is useful to counter the catabolic effect of elevated cortisol. As part of a pre- and post-workout protocol, glutamine is a nutrient that is not to be ignored.

Effective Dose: As supported in studies, look to provide a range from 15 - 30 g/day which may be divided in a pre and post dose.

Nucleotides – Often neglected in many pre- and post-workout supplements, nucleotides are the building blocks of all genetic material (DNA & RNA). They also play critical roles in supporting immune function, GI health and muscle repair (more about this in chapter 5). When your resistance is low and the body is fighting viral or bacterial infections, your immune system must create new, quickly functioning immune cells and antibodies. As old cells die, new ones must be created, which require an adequate nucleotide supply. When tissues or organs have been damaged, new cells must take their place. The immune system and gastrointestinal tract (the largest immune organ in the body) are dependent on nucleotides for rapid immune cell growth and repair. Emerging evidence suggests that dietary nucleotides optimize immune function by influencing the development, activation and proliferation of immune cells such as lymphocytes and macrophages. They stimulate antibody production and increase resistance to infections. In fact, they are needed in greater quantities during recovery and periods of stress and infection and may even reduce cortisol levels after intense exercise. As part of a pre- and post-workout protocol, nucleotides are an important component for both immune and muscle maintenance.

Effective Dose: As supported in studies, look to supply 500 mg - 1,000 mg which may be divided in a pre and post dose

Immune Peptides in Whey Protein Isolates/Concentrates – While whey has taken center stage as a superior protein source among sports supplements, it's also rich in compounds called immune peptides that support immune health. They include beta-lactoglobulin, alpha-lactalbumin, immunoglobulins (IgGs), glycomacropeptides, bovine serum albumin, and minor peptides such as lactoperoxidases, lysozyme and lactoferrin. Immune peptides are known to enhance the production and activity of many immune components for defense, antimicrobial and anti-inflammatory effects. Lactoferrin, for example, is an important first line of defense against several viruses by binding to receptors on viruses and preventing them from infecting healthy cells. Whey protein also helps maintain a healthy immune system because of its high biological value, high levels of branch chain amino acids and its ability to increase glutathione levels in the body. Glutathione is an important antioxidant for immune support. You will not find immune peptides in any other protein nor the biological value whey possesses. For these reasons, it is the ideal protein for building muscle and supporting immune function. More on this in chapter five.

Effective Dose: Add 20 g – 30 g of whey protein (isolate or concentrate) to your daily post workout beverage. In addition, after calculating your total protein needs (chapter 6), supplement your diet in this dosage range to satisfy your daily protein requirements if needed.

Probiotics – Probiotics are the "friendly" bacteria that reside in the gastrointestinal (GI) tract and play a vital role in immunity and GI health. They are found in fermented foods such as yogurt and tempeh. Different strains colonize different parts of the intestines. Important to the health of the body are strains such as *Lactobacillus* (e.g. *L. acidophilus*) that live in the upper GI tract and *Bifidobacteria* (e.g. *B. bifidus*) that calls the lower intestines home. Since your GI tract is the largest immune organ in the body, these beneficial bacteria play an important part in immune health by: normalizing GI defenses, reducing inflammation, crowding out "bad" bacteria, assisting in detoxification, and producing natural antibiotics.

Effective Dose: Look for probiotic products that provide at least 1 – 5 billion viable organisms and have a blend of both *Lactobacillus* and *Bifido* bacteria strains. Make sure they are either refrigerated or shelf stable products – in either case, refrigerate at home.

Beta 1,3/1,6 Glucans – beta glucans are carbohydrate polymers (polysaccharides) typically derived from the cell walls of yeast, oats, barley, and mushrooms. Specifically, the form of beta glucans most studied for immune enhancement is the beta-1,3/1,6 glucans from yeast. Along with beta 1,4 glucans from oats, the yeast form has also been shown to exhibit protective cardiovascular effects by reducing bad LDL cholesterol. There are numerous research papers on the immune-enhancing effects of beta 1,3/1,6 glucans, including stimulating the activity of white blood cells, macrophage, and natural killer cells (all of which are suppressed by intense exercise). Beta 1,3/1,6 glucans increase the number, size and function of certain immune cells while enhancing total immune defense. Known as biological defense modifiers, they are able to bind to immune cells and directly activate their function. Research has demonstrated that 200mg of regular beta 1,3/1,6 glucans or as little as 7 - 10 mg of a highly purified beta-1,3/1,6 glucan form is sufficient to activate an immune response.

Effective Dose: As supported in studies, look to supply either 200mg or 7 - 10 mg daily of a highly purified beta 1,3/1,6 glucans on training days.

Honorable Mention: L-arginine – the amino acid L-arginine plays important roles in protein synthesis, production of nitric oxide, removing ammonia from the body, and influences growth hormone and insulin. Aside from its ability to influence growth hormone, L-arginine is an important amino acid that exerts positive effects on immune function by increasing the activity of natural killer cells and helps regulate the activity of the thymus gland, which is responsible for manufacturing T-cells. Medically, it has been used in high-risk surgical patients to improve immune response and increase resistance to infections. Effective levels include 3 – 5g daily.

Supplements for Anti-inflammatory Support

Omega-3 Fish Oils – Out of all the fats in the diet, omega-3 polyunsaturated fatty acids (PUFA) have the most significant immune-modulating effects. When we speak of omega-3, we really are referring to the two important fatty acids eicosapentaenoic acid (EPA) and docosahexaenoic acid (DHA). Research shows that omega-3 fatty acids reduce inflammation and may lower the risk of degenerative diseases, such as cardiovascular disease, cancer, and arthritis. They do this by inhibiting the production of prostaglandins, hormone-like substances that regulate many physiological functions including blood pressure, blood clotting, nerve transmission, and the inflammatory and allergic responses. Unfortunately, Americans consume too much polyunsaturated omega-6 fats found in vegetable oils such as corn and canola. High intakes of omega-6 fats have the opposite effect on prostaglandins as compared to omega-3 fats. That is, they *promote* the release of prostaglandins that cause inflammation. Therefore, efforts must be made to replace some of the omega-6 fats in your diet with omega-3 fats to help keep inflammation under control. Omega-3 fats seem to have the same effect during intense exercise where there is increased production of inflammatory messengers. Studies also show that when omega-3 fats are combined with antioxidants, muscle recovery is enhanced and inflammation is lowered.

Effective Dose: As supported in studies, look to supply 1 - 3 g of EPA and DHA daily - dosing for fish oil supplements should be based on the amount of EPA and DHA, not on the total amount of fish oil.

Vitamin C– perhaps the most well-known and researched antioxidant vitamin, vitamin C deserves a mention here because of its effect on inflammatory messengers, especially cortisol. As we discussed, chronic elevated cortisol is implicated in muscle breakdown and decreased immune function. Several studies examining the effects of vitamin C during both endurance and resistance exercise show a positive effect on lowering this menacing hormone. When marathon runners were supplemented with vitamin C, lower circulating concentrations of cortisol and other inflammatory markers were observed. In weight lifters, consumption of 1 - 2 g of vitamin C was also shown to lower cortisol levels. Interestingly, other studies show that lower doses of vitamins C are also helpful for reducing muscle soreness and improving muscle function.

Effective Dose: As supported in studies, look to supply 1 – 3 gm daily which may be divided in a pre and post dose.

Phosphatidylserine (PS) – a lipid derivative that's important to many aspects of cellular functioning and communication, phosphatidylserine may play a role in modulating the stress response and cortisol levels as well. Studies indicate that phosphatidylserine supplementation can potentially lower serum cortisol in response to acute exercise stress in a dose-dependent fashion. Short-term supplementation with a moderate dose of 600 mg – 750 mg per day after intense activity in healthy males was shown to effectively reduce exercise-induced stress by blunting the rise in cortisol levels and reducing muscle soreness after exercise. Additional studies demonstrate the ability of PS to improve exercise capacity during high-intensity cycling and tended to increase performance during intermittent running competition.

Effective Dose: As supported in studies, look to supply 600 – 750 mg daily.

Boswellia Resin Extract – the *Boswellia serrata* plant has been used in traditional Indian medicine for centuries and contains active components that inhibit the cyclooxygenase-2 (COX2) and 5-lipoxygenase enzyme pathways. These enzymes play a key role in promoting the inflammatory response. The brand 5-Loxin® is an enriched extract from *Boswellia* that contains 30% 3-O-acetyl-11-keto-beta-boswellic acid (AKBA), the most potent of the boswellic acids for inhibiting 5-lipoxygenase. Its effect on the inflammatory 5-lipoxygenase enzyme and the cartilage-degrading metalloproteinase enzyme was studied in 75 subjects with osteoarthritis using 100 mg or 250 mg for 90 days. Both doses resulted in statistically significant improvements in mobility and reducing the negative effects of these enzymes. Other studies demonstrate significant safety profiles of *Boswellia* and its component 5-Loxin®.

Effective Dose: As supported in studies, look for the trademarked 5-Loxin® *Boswellia* product – 100 to 250 mg daily if needed.

Turmeric Root Extract– from the plant *Curcuma longa*, turmeric has been used for thousands of years to treat a variety of ailments. In several studies, turmeric's active components, most notably curcuminoids, have demonstrated potent anti-inflammatory effects in patients with osteoarthritis when compared to drugs, such as hydrocortisone, phenylbutazone and Motrin (Ibuprofen) without side effects commonly seen with these drugs. Curcuminoids inhibit the breakdown of arachidonic acid, a potent pro-inflammatory fatty acid, and decreases the activity of inflammatory messengers from the immune system. In one animal study, administration of curcuminoids was shown to reduce the inflammatory cytokines and offset some of the performance deficits associated with inflammation and exercise-induced muscle damage. Look for extracts standardized for curcuminoids.

Effective Dose: As supported in studies, look to supply at least 400 mg of a standardized extract 2-3 times daily if needed.

CHAPTER 3
Exercise and Oxidative Stress:
How Free Radicals Break You Down

Without oxygen we cannot survive and because of it we will surely die. It is also critical for the production of adenosine triphosphate (ATP), the energy molecule that drives all chemical and physiological activites in the body. In the wake of energy production, however, byproducts called free radicals - highly reactive molecules that attack cellular components - are created and implicated as the cause of disease and even the aging process itself. Yet, despite their infamy, free radicals can benefit the body. They are an important part of the immune response by certain cells that produce free

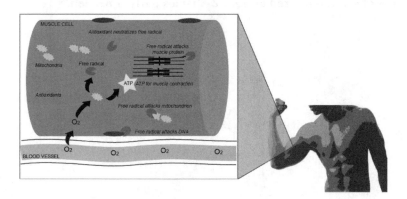

radicals as a weapon against viruses and bacteria. Some free radicals are used as signaling molecules to turn on and off cellular functions. Left unchecked, however, they would wreak biochemical havoc in every cell in the body. In addition, the more oxygen consumed for energy production, the potential for increased free-radical production. Nowhere is this more apparent than during strenuous activity as working muscles require more and more oxygen to produce ATP and sustain activity. Additionally, as discussed in chapter two, the presence of inflammation that arises as a result of strenuous activity can further free-radical production also known as "oxidative stress". Unfortunate for the athlete, the build-up and/or poor clearance of free radicals is a significant contributor to fatigue, muscle breakdown, and prolonged recovery.

Increased oxidative stress can be seen within a short period of time after exercise and initiate the release of inflammatory cytokines (as discussed in chapter two) contributing to further damage. This has been documented in several studies where markers of oxidative stress are elevated following strenuous exercise. Endurance exercise increases oxygen utilization well above the resting state and significantly increases free-radical production. So important is it to quench free radicals that the body has developed several antioxidant mechanisms.

Free–radical production increases during strenuous exercise and if left unchecked can increase muscle fatigue & breakdown, prolong recovery, as well as decrease physical performance.

The body's antioxidant defenses are classified into two groups: dietary antioxidants and endogenous antioxidants. Dietary antioxidants include vitamins A, C, and E, minerals such as selenium, zinc, copper, and manganese and a host of plant-based antioxidants such as the class of polyphenols. They contribute to the antioxidant reserve yet play only a secondary role to the body's internal intracellular antioxidant systems. Endogenous antioxidants are the critical components that all cells produce to defend against free radicals. They include superoxide dismutase (SOD), catalase and glutathione peroxidase and represent the most powerful line of defense against oxidative stress. Table one summarizes the major endogenous antioxidant systems and a further description is provided in the subsequent paragraphs.

Table 1. Major antioxidant systems in the body's tissues used to combat oxidative stress

Antioxidant System	Physiological Function	Reaction summary
Glutathione Glutathione Peroxidase (GPx) Glutathione Reductase (GRed)	Glutathione is a two-residue amino acid (cysteine and glutamate) antioxidant that breaks down hydrogen peroxide into water. **Selenium** acts as a cofactor for GPx **Vitamin B$_2$** (specifically FAD) is a cofactor for GRed Note: this system is dietary-enhanced with **N-acetyl cysteine**	Glutathione-SH Glutathione-SH H2O2 Hydrogen Peroxide (↑ Ox. Stress) GRed GPx Glutathione-S-S-Glutathione H2O Water
Superoxide Dismutase (SOD) Peroxiredoxins Catalase	With the help of catalase, **SOD** breaks down superoxide into water. **Copper** and **zinc** are cofactors for cytosolic SODs **Manganese** is a cofactor for mitochondrial SODs	Mitochondrial Respiration SOD Peroxiredoxins Catalase $O_2 \longrightarrow {}^{\bullet}O_2^{-} \longrightarrow H_2O_2 \longrightarrow H_2O$ Oxygen Superoxide (↑ Ox. Stress) Hydrogen Peroxide (↑ Ox. Stress) Water

Out of all the endogenous antioxidants, SOD is perhaps the most important because it neutralizes a form of oxygen called superoxide radical. So biologically toxic is this free radical that every cell in the body must produce SOD to survive. Since its discovery in 1968, SOD has held great interest in the medical field. Its primary function is to convert superoxide into a less harmful compound for other antioxidants (i.e., catalase and glutathione) to eliminate. But it also plays other important roles including support of the immune system and reducing inflammatory cytokines, which are altered during strenuous exercise. Remember, the production of free radicals during intense activity cannot be curtailed, but their activity and longevity can. That is the function of antioxidants: to reduce the amounts and activity of free radicals as soon as possible. The more antioxidants available, the more efficient the system and the better the body becomes at controlling inflammation and supporting performance and recovery.

The concerns for every athlete are: to what extent the athlete is prepared for this barrage of free radicals, how effective can the athlete defend against free radicals, and do they need to take extra antioxidants? This is where proper diet plays an important role. Poor nutritional status cannot compensate for the free radicals generated during high-intensity exercise and increased oxygen intake. The result is oxidative stress. Diet, antioxidant intake, and rest must be considered to prevent muscle pain and tenderness after activity and reduce inflammation, swelling, and loss of strength.

How Much of a Concern for the Athlete? First, The Good News

There is no doubt that regular, moderate exercise does a world of good for the body – from athletic performance to disease prevention. Many studies demonstrate the efficacy of mild to moderate exercise for heart disease, osteoporosis and diabetes. In fact, numerous studies show that moderate exercise stimulates endogenous antioxidant systems to adapt to oxidative stress more efficiently. Simple dietary modification, proper nutrition supplements, and adequate rest will positively affect antioxidant status and immune function during strenuous activity. Athletes must maintain a well-balanced diet rich in vitamins, minerals and phytonutrients that support antioxidant defenses and strive for at least eight hours of sleep.

Now, The Bad News

While muscles respond positively to moderate exercise (i.e., increasing the production of endogenous antioxidants), free radicals produced during intense exercise can exceed antioxidant defenses that may be marginal because of poor nutritional status. At the microscopic level, excessive free radicals cause significant disruption to DNA, enzymes, and cell membrane structures inside muscles, resulting in fatigue, soreness and prolonged recovery. Just think of the casual runner participating in a marathon and the ensuing muscle soreness that occurs. Untrained and older athletes or "weekend warriors" are more susceptible to exercise-induced free radical damage and prolonged recovery. So, while endurance training supports physiological adaptation to exercise, constantly training at high levels eventually compromises the body's antioxidant defenses.

Strenuous physical activity greatly increases oxygen consumption to meet energy demands, which creates a state of "oxidative stress" that can increase cardiovascular risk.

In addition to affecting muscle performance and recovery, free radicals can narrow bronchial airways and reduce lung function. One study showed that one in three college athletes may have a condition called "exercise-induced asthma" or "exercise-induced bronchoconstriction," even without any history of breathing difficulties. Researchers have attributed this effect to increased free-radical production after intense exercise as the culprit by eliciting an immune response and constricting the airways due to inflammation. One way to act in a preventative fashion is to adopt an anti-inflammatory diet and use of omega-3 fatty acids [eicosapentaenoic acid (EPA) and docosahexaenoic acid (DHA)]. Several papers have been published on their beneficial role in reducing exercise-induced asthma. Briefly, omega-3 fatty acids act by competing with components needed for the formation of inflammatory compounds (leukotrienes and prostaglandins) responsible for the constriction of airways.

If it were only possible to stop breathing, you could avoid free radical–production and oxidative stress all together! A more practical, and safer, approach is to enhance the antioxidant defenses of the body through proper diet and supplementation.

Nutritional Support: The Antioxidant Arsenal

In addition to the anti-inflammatory diet and supplement regimen suggested in chapter two, nutritional strategies to combat oxidative stress are necessary. A diet rich in fruits and vegetables that supply many key antioxidant nutrients is the starting point. Avoiding fructose (including high-fructose corn syrup) is strongly recommended since it has been implicated in insulin resistance, atherosclerosis, and obesity. New data shows that fructose, which is found in many sports drinks and protein supplements, can actually contribute to oxidative stress. A recent study reported that fructose added to a preworkout beverage can significantly increase oxidative stress as compared to beverages without fructose. Supplementing with antioxidants and supporting the endogenous antioxidant enzymes (catalase, SOD, and glutathione peroxidase) is used in conjunction with dietary modification. Dietary antioxidants include:

- vitamins A, C, and E
- minerals such as zinc, copper, and manganese
- nutraceuticals including carotenoids, tocotrienols, coenzyme Q10, alpha lipoic acid, and n-acetyl-cysteine
- phytonutrients and flavonoids found in green tea, grape skin, pine bark, and citrus fruits

Avoid beverages containing fructose or high-fructose corn syrup (HCFS). New data reveals that when added to a pre-workout drink, this "bad" sugar can trigger oxidative stress – something an athlete certainly does not need!

A review of the literature shows that diets rich in phytonutrient antioxidants (found abundantly in dark colored fruits and vegetables) provide superior antioxidant protection against exercise-induced oxidative stress. Unfortunately, getting most people to eat the recommended five to seven servings of fruits and vegetables daily is a challenge. In a culture where convenience is king and a burger and fries costs less than a bag of carrots, most people do not eat properly. It is especially important for athletes to consider additional nutritional requirements as their needs are increased for several nutrients above and beyond that which can be supplied by diet alone. Some researchers contend that chronic strenuous exercise may create a state of oxidative stress whereby endogenous antioxidant enzymes are unable to ward off. For this reason, supplementation is warranted. This is especially true for endurance athletes whose increased oxygen and energy demands predispose them to oxidative stress. Before starting or continuing an exercise regimen, nutritional and antioxidant status should be determined.

Deficiency of antioxidant nutrients can augment exercise-induced oxidative stress. Some research now suggests that supplementation of specific dietary antioxidants may be extremely beneficial for those involved in strenuous activity.

It is important to stress that this book does not advocate a "magic bullet" approach to supplementation. To think that protein supplements alone or high doses of vitamin C will enhance performance is myopic at best. Vitamins, minerals, and antioxidants are not isolated components in the body but rather, an integrated system working synergistically. Therefore, a full array of both fat- and water-soluble nutrients and antioxidants is the best defense against oxidative stress. Lastly, it is imperative that you understand the role antioxidants play in protecting the body against oxidative stress. They are not meant to make you jump higher or run faster. Rather, antioxidants found in foods and supplements mitigate the effects of intense exercise (i.e. oxidative stress and inflammation) and thus, support the body's natural ability to recover. It is also important not to focus on the short term benefits of antioxidants, but rather focus on the long-term protective effects in conditions associated with depressed defenses. Remember, it is recovery that makes the body stronger and if we view the athlete as a patient under stress, then treating this condition with a whole host of dietary and endogenous antioxidants is the most prudent course of action. Specific recommendations for the type and amounts of antioxidant nutrients vary from person to person and should be determined by a certified or licensed sports nutritionist.

The Antioxidant Players

The first line of antioxidant defense begins within the fat-soluble cellular membranes of the cell. Here, vitamin E (both tocopherols and tocotrienols), beta-carotene (and other carotenoids), lipoic acid, coenzyme Q10, and numerous polyphenols found in fruits and tea are the major players. For example, antioxidant rich extracts of blueberries have been shown to counter the damage to muscle cells exposed to free radicals in-vitro since they are rich in potent antioxidants that include phenolics acids, tannins, flavonols and anthocyanins – all part of the polyphenol family. Within the cell, the water-soluble antioxidant vitamin C and the endogenous antioxidant enzymes (glutathione peroxidase, SOD, and catalase) dominate. Again, consuming nutrient rich foods is the primary route for dietary antioxidants. Only when the diet is lacking (which is often the case) is supplementation warranted. Endogenous antioxidants aren't typically found in high concentrations in foods and must be supplemented. There is no concern that supplemental antioxidant therapy with endogenous antioxidants will override the body's antioxidant defense and cause negative effects. The preponderance of the research suggests taking supplemental antioxidants augments the endogenous antioxidants systems – serving to fill the battle voids in the war against oxidative stress.

There are numerous antioxidant and anti-inflammatory compounds in many fruits as well as extracts of green/black tea, red wine, chocolate, pine bark, grape seed/skin and cherries that play important roles in reducing free-radical damage caused by exercise-induced oxidative stress.

The Endogenous Players

Superoxide Dismutase (SOD) – SOD was first used as an injectable form to treat arthritis, reduce inflammation, relieve asthma, and used as an adjunctive cancer therapy. In addition, SOD has found its place as an important player in immune and cardiovascular health. SOD's primary function is to convert the free radical, superoxide, into a less harmful hydrogen peroxide molecule for subsequent dismantling by glutathione and catalase. While SOD is a critical antioxidant for all cells of the body, diet alone does not supply appreciable levels. Since SOD is a protein, it is easily destroyed in the digestive tract and rendered clinically useless. Recently, however, an orally effective form is available under the trademark GliSODin®. This form has been the subject of several published clinical trials in humans demonstrating remarkable immune, anti-inflammatory and antioxidant effects. Studies clearly show that taking GliSODin® for two weeks protected healthy individuals against oxidative stress when exposed to hyperbaric oxygen, reduced lactate and free-radical accumulation in cyclists after intense training, and improved arterial function by reducing the thickness of the carotid artery (an indicator of cardiovascular disease).

Effective Dose: Studies support 250 - 500 mg GliSODin® daily

Glutathione – glutathione is comprised of the amino acids glycine, glutamate, and cysteine. In its reduced form (GSH), it is a major intracellular antioxidant. Glutathione is well known for its significant role as an antioxidant and detoxifying agent: not only neutralizing free radicals but eliminating toxins as well. Its protective role comes at a cost as GSH levels can quickly decline as a consequence of neutralizing free radicals and toxins. One of the most reliable ways to assess oxidative stress from exercise is to measure the breakdown of glutathione, which can be rapid. Low levels are implicated in a variety of diseases such as cancer, neurodegenerative and immuno-compromised conditions. Several studies in endurance athletes have shown decreased plasma levels after exercise, indicating an increased utilization and need in working muscles. Glutathione, like SOD, is difficult to absorb as a dietary supplement. While some intact glutathione may pass through the intestinal wall, most of it will be degraded by digestive enzymes. Nevertheless, the by-products of digestion yield important building blocks required for glutathione's production. One supplement that has been shown to effectively and safely increase glutathione synthesis is N-acetyl cysteine (NAC). Coupling glutathione with other antioxidants, like alpha lipoic acid, preserves its levels by recycling spent glutathione and reducing exercise-induced glutathione breakdown.

Effective Dose: If taking a glutathione, 150 mg per day from a reputable source such as the trademarked glutathione from Kyowa Hakko called Setria®. Since intact glutathione absorption is limited, antioxidants like lipoic acid and NAC are recommended as well.

The Exogenous Players – A Select Few

Vitamin C & Vitamin E – entire books have been written about the vitamins A, C, and E as well as the minerals zinc, selenium, copper, and manganese. All of these play pivotal roles in supporting antioxidant systems in the body. They have been extensively studied for their role in reducing oxidative stress during strenuous exercise. Several studies have investigated the ability of vitamins C and E to reduce exercise-induced oxidative stress and support the immune system. Interestingly, the subjects who received vitamin C and E exhibited reduced oxidative stress without interfering with the normal adaptation to exercise. Other studies have shown that vitamin C alone can help reduce muscle soreness, delay muscle breakdown and support antioxidant protection. Also, studies have demonstrated a protective effect against exercise-induced airway narrowing in asthmatic subjects when given vitamin C. Most recently, vitamins C and E were shown to support antioxidant defenses in basketball players undergoing strenuous training and competition.

Effective Dose: studies support 500 mg to 1.5 g of vitamin C and 200 IU to 400 IU of vitamin E daily.

Alpha Lipoic Acid and NAC – we have briefly described how NAC supports glutathione levels. In addition, NAC has been shown to have a protective effect on the lungs during increased respiration and may help reduce fatigue during strenuous activity. Alpha lipoic acid (a.k.a. lipoic acid) is a hydrocarbon-rich, sulfur-containing antioxidant compound. Other sulfur based antioxidants include cysteine, methionine, taurine and N-acetylcysteine (NAC). In a comparison to various forms of lipoic acid, R-lipoic acid (the reduced form of alpha lipoic acid) is the most effective. Besides its role as a direct antioxidant, lipoic acid also maintains a healthy antioxidant network by regenerating glutathione, vitamin C, and vitamin E. Studies of subjects undergoing resistance training showed that when given 600 mg of alpha lipoic acid daily, glutathione levels increased and, markers of oxidative stress were reduced. This protective effect is critical for all athletes. Lipoic acid also reduces exercise-induced declines in SOD activity while also increasing catalase activity. When combined with NAC, they are more effective at increasing total antioxidant status and reducing oxidative stress after exercise.

Effective Dose: Studies support 600 mg of R-lipoic acid daily. For NAC, studies support 600 mgs two to three times daily.

Green/Black Tea Extracts – prepared from the leaves of *Camellia sinensis*, green and black tea is particularly concentrated in phytonutrients including polyphenols, flavonoids, and the well-studied catechins. The most potent of the catechins is epigallocatechin-3-gallate (EGCG). The antioxidant activity of EGCG is about 25 to 100 times more potent than vitamins C and E. One cup of green tea provides 10 mg to 40 mg of polyphenols and has a greater antioxidant effect than a serving of broccoli or strawberries. Green tea reduces several markers of oxidative stress (e.g., concentrations of lipid peroxides were reduced while glutathione was increased) and influences indicators of muscle breakdown after strenuous exercise. A particular constituent found in black tea, called theaflavins, has also been found to reduce oxidative stress via its role as an antioxidant and anti-inflammatory agent. Several in-vitro studies have confirmed this phytonutrient to exert potent effects on gene expression related to inflammation. In response to acute, high-intensity exercise, theaflavins helped to increase performance parameters and reduce muscle soreness.

Effective Dose: studies support 300 - 400 mg green tea extract (standardized for EGCG) or black tea extract (standardized for theaflavins).

Tart Cherry - it is well known that tart cherries have a significant amount of polyphenols, which we have already established as having powerful antioxidant properties. Interestingly, consumption of about 45 cherries per day has been shown to reduce inflammatory markers in healthy men and a woman while other studies demonstrated cherry's ability to decrease C-reactive protein. With respect to athletes, increasing cherry consumption to approximately 100 per day reduces the loss of strength following exercise-induced muscle damage. A recent study of long distance runners given tart cherry juice for seven days had significantly reduced pain after training, signifying reduced inflammation and free-radical production.

Effective Dose: Studies support approximately 100 cherries daily or approximately two 10 ounces to 12 ounces tart cherry juice containing a standardized amount of phenolic compounds or 1,200 mg of standardized cherry extract

CHAPTER 4
Exercise, Fatigue and Energy Production

Have you ever "hit the wall?" Tired, worn out or exhausted and just cannot get in that last effort? Fatigue is defined as an inability to function and do work due to a lack of energy. Every athlete experiences fatigue and achieving optimum performance requires the ability to produce cellular energy (adenosine triphosphate (ATP)) efficiently, effectively clear metabolic waste by-products (i.e., lactic acid, free radicals, inflammatory markers) and recover quicly before the next training. The frequency and extent of fatigue depends upon several factors including diet and supplement regimen, training techniques, stress level, and the amount of sleep. All of these factors, along with genetics, will determine how well the body produces and sustains energy and work output.

We marvel at the efficiency of the human machine and how it can adapt to exercise. Within every cell are minute energy producing powerhouses called mitochondria whose sole purpose is to produce ATP. Exercise stimulates the function and increases the number of mitochondria (known as "mitochondrial biogenesis"). Within a week of hard training, the body is able to generate energy more efficiently, do more work, and prevent fatigue. The most dramatic clinical cases of fatigue I have seen are with immune-compromised conditions such as cancer and AIDS. Depending upon the study, fatigue can occur in up to 95 percent of oncology patients as a consequence of the disease and treatment. On a cellular level, the fatigue seen in these groups is the result of inflammation, reduced lactate clearance, damage to the mitochondria and disruption of normal energy metabolism. *This same process occurs during and after strenuous exercise and has the same effect as seen in disease states.* While fatigue is a very complex biological, neurological, and physiological process, the ability to deal with it boils down to the reserves of energy stored in muscle and the ability to produce energy in the mitochondria efficiently regardless of whether it is a cancer patient or elite athlete. This is especially true of the athlete who consistently overtrains and taxes his/her body beyond their capacity.

Energy Production

To make muscles work, energy from food (calories) must be converted in mitochondria to the chemical form of cellular energy called adenosine triphosphate (ATP). It is the mitochondria that act like batteries inside every cell, producing ATP that serves as the currency for all energy needs of the body. Adenosine triphosphate is a very simple molecule comprised of an adenosine molecule, ribose, and three phosphate molecules. Regardless of the type of exercise, the ability to perform work is based upon adequate and efficient production of ATP inside muscles. The more mitochondria packed into a muscle, the more work the muscle can do, whether it is hitting a tennis ball, lifting weights or running a marathon. In addition to intensity, the duration of exercise also affects ATP metabolism: the shorter the time of activity, the more the muscle depends on immediate stores of ATP.

Chronic fatigue is a common response to intense activity (70 – 90% maximal heart rate) for extended periods of time. During intense activity, the demands for ATP may outpace its production and result in decreased exercise performance.

One of the primary fuels used to produce ATP is glucose, which is derived from carbohydrates in food or pulled from stores in the liver and muscle (called "glycogen"). Through the process called "glycolysis", glucose is released from storage and provided to cells for energy production. Storage of glucose in the liver and muscles allows the body to maintain an even supply of glucose despite fluctuations in the diet. If these stores did not exist, energy production would be jeopardized. However, the body is capable of producing glucose from other sources including protein from muscle or fat. The production of energy in the cell occurs either in the presence of oxygen (called "aerobic respiration") or in its absence ("anaerobic respiration"). Aerobic respiration is preferred because ATP production is most efficient - approximately 20 times more than without oxygen. The heart, kidneys, liver, and muscles rely heavily on aerobic respiration. To meet the demands of intense exercise, the cell relies on producing both new ATP and regenerating spent ATP – a process known as "oxidative phosphorylation." During energy production ATP loses a phosphate group, releasing energy, and leaving behind the molecule adenosine diphosphate (ADP). So important is ATP that even spent ADP is conserved and converted back to ATP. These biochemical processes are critical for continuous energy production in working muscles.

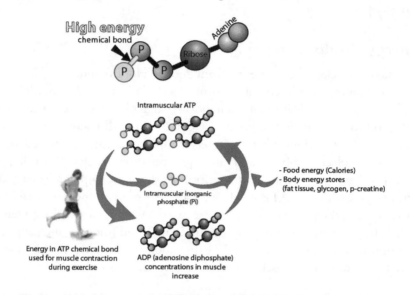

Compounds like creatine are needed for efficient ATP production and regeneration. Creatine is produced in several organs including the liver and kidneys and converts to creatine phosphate (CP) in the mitochondria. Its availability to muscle cells is influenced by the hormone insulin and dietary intake of carbohydrates. Yes, carbohydrates help increase the absorption and uptake of creatine! As creatine phosphate, it is an energy shuttle in the cell and very capable of supporting the conversion of ADP back to ATP. As activity revs up, creatine phosphate stores are immediately mobilized for muscles to meet the demands for increased workloads. The more intense the activity, the quicker the stores are depleted, requiring the body to quickly shift from aerobic metabolism (generating a lot of energy via oxygen) to anaerobic metabolism (generating less energy without the use of oxygen).

In addition to producing less ATP, anaerobic metabolism produces more lactic acid and hydrogen ions. Often felt as a "burn," increased lactic acid and hydrogen ions acidify muscle tissue and decrease performance. So, an ample supply of glucose or other energy substrates, creatine, nucleotides (adenosine), and ribose with an adequate supply of oxygen is the ideal scenario to optimize muscle activity. This is not an easy task when the activity gets progressively intense or prolonged. While muscle activity prefers a steady supply of ATP from glucose, exercising for extended periods requires other sources for energy production: fat (as free fatty acids) and potentially protein. Which fuel source the body chooses depends on the nutritional state of the individual and the intensity and duration of activity. Carbohydrate stores supply ATP production for approximately 90 minutes of constant physical activity, while fat stores may last several days. However, obtaining energy from fat and protein is not as efficient as from carbohydrates and, in the case of protein, may actually lead to muscle breakdown. Case in point: researchers in the early 1980's determined that starved cyclists break down muscle protein during prolonged cycling and this effect was completely blunted when carbohydrates were given prior to the same exercise.

Fatigue: Is It All In your Head!

The subject of exercise fatigue is rather complex since it involves a number of factors that all play an important part in its development. These include nutritional state, level of hydration, training techniques, genetics, exercise type and intensity, heat exposure, availability of energy substrates, excess protein intake, and acidosis. From a very basic level, most fatigue associated with exercise involves some degree of both peripheral and central fatigue. Peripheral fatigue deals with the capacity of muscles to do work in response to nerve signals from the brain. Those signals can be disrupted during intense exercise for a variety of reasons including increased lactic acid levels, diminishing ATP levels, and accumulation of free radicals. It is interesting to note that peripheral fatigue is seen in immune-compromised patients and most likely results from the same mechanisms that occur during strenuous exercise. Central fatigue involves the connections between the brain and network of nerves found in muscle tissue. Alterations in neurotransmitters, like acetylcholine and serotonin, may be the cause of central fatigue.

Carbohydrates and a proper carbohydrate-to-protein ratio are essential for muscle performance. When glycogen stores in the muscle are exhausted and dietary carbohydrates are insufficient to replenish those stores, the body will break down muscle and use protein for energy production. Protein is composed of amino acids and falling blood levels of amino acid (because of their use as energy substrates) contribute to fatigue. For example, low blood levels of branch chain amino acids (valine, leucine, and isoleucine) may increase the entry of another amino acid – tryptophan – into the brain. Elevated tryptophan leads to increased production of the neurotransmitter serotonin that contributes to the feeling of fatigue. New data suggests that serotonin is not the only neurotransmitter involved and that dopamine and norepinephrine play a part as well. Studies suggest that an increase of the serotonin-to-dopamine ratio is associated with feelings of tiredness and accelerates fatigue, while others suggest a role for dopamine and norepinephrine influencing exercise performance. So, while there has been a lot of discussion about lactic acid as a cause of fatigue, imbalances in neurotransmitter levels may play a comparable, if not greater, role in exercise-induced fatigue.

Potential Energy Players

As with all supplements, their use needs to be weighed against the data that exists and are secondary to diet and training. Nevertheless, interesting findings may warrant their short-term use for the competitive athlete.

Creatine – while the next chapter discusses how creatine positively influences strength and performance, many of the studies also show evidence of creatine improving short-term exercise performance when combined with resistance exercise. In addition, emerging data suggests that creatine can support brain health. Studies have demonstrated that creatine has a regulatory role on improving ATP production in the brain and adequate creatine levels may improve memory and reduce mental fatigue. In a study that combined creatine with the antioxidant alpha lipoic acid, greater concentrations of creatine phosphate were found in muscles. Taken together, the anabolic effects of creatine supplementation may now be coupled with its ability to positively affect mental performance and reduce fatigue – an effect most interesting to athletes!
Effective Dose: Studies support 3 g to 5 g per day (may be divided equally for pre and post workout).

Nucleotides – Nucleotides are found everywhere within the cells of the body and some, such as cyclic adenosine monophosphate (cAMP) serve as critical cellular messengers. Others serve as the structural units that make up cellular components, including adenosine triphosphate. Nucleotides are considered conditionally essential (a nutrient that must be supplied by diet or supplementation under special conditions like stress or illness) and promote protein synthesis during periods of stress, rapid growth, and tissue repair. Serious consideration needs to be given to nucleotides for the athlete during and after intense training or competition when regeneration of ATP requires sufficient nucleotide levels. Most studies using supplemental nucleotides have been limited to liver and gastrointestinal disorders as well as playing an important role in immunity and tissue repair. Animal studies have confirmed that dietary nucleotides help restore mitochondrial function and improve energy production. Researchers suggest supplementing with nucleotides can act as precursors in the synthesis of mitochondrial DNA and ATP and assist in rapid normalization of mitochondrial function. Studies in the athletic population are needed, but being conditionally essential nutrients during stressful conditions warrants their use in the athlete.

Effective Dose: Studies support 200 - 500 mg daily.

Carnitine – carnitine (also called L-carnitine) is synthesized in the liver and kidneys from the amino acids lysine and methionine. For athletes, an important role carnitine serves is to release stored fat (fatty acids) and transport them into the mitochondria for energy production. In this way, it supports energy levels during long-term aerobic activity. Studies in athletes have shown that carnitine supplementation can positively affect performance by increasing muscle oxygen consumption and stimulating fat metabolism for energy use. Carnitine has also been shown to reduce the hypoxic (oxygen deprived) effects of extended periods of exercise, lower lactic acid production, and speed up recovery. The use of 1 - 2 g of Carnipure® (L-carnitine-L-tartrate) in athletes and healthy subjects confirmed these effects by showing less tissue damage, reduced muscle soreness, and quicker recovery.

Effective Dose: Studies support 1 – 2g daily taken away from meals - you do not want carnitine to compete for absorption with amino acids from dietary protein.

L-Alanyl-L-glutamine (AlaGln) – this compound consists of two amino acids (l-alanine and l-glutamine), both of which support energy production separately. Glutamine can be used as a direct substrate for energy production, stimulates protein synthesis and wound healing, and supports immune function. L-alanine helps rebuild glycogen stores. When bonded together, AlaGln can promote muscle rehydration. Dehydration is a major cause of fatigue in athletes and only small deficits can result in decreased performance. L-alanyl-L-glutamine helps absorb water and electrolytes in the intestinal tract. A recent study showed that AlaGln increases performance in endurance athletes by preventing dehydration during exercise. Water alone did not appear to significantly offset the performance reduction.

Effective Dose: Studies support a dose of 50 mg per kilogram body weight. Look for a reputable source of AlaGln such as Sustamine®.

Branch Chain Amino Acids (BCAAs) - along with fatty acids, branch chain amino acids are valuable energy sources for ATP production when glycogen levels are low. In addition, BCAAs have the ability to combat central fatigue since they compete for tryptophan in the brain, which prevents increased levels of serotonin (a neurotransmitter that makes you tired). For endurance athletes, the use of BCAAs before and after the workout has shown to be effective in delaying the time to fatigue and improve mental performance. In addition to these effects, some studies have demonstrated a reduction in lactic acid and muscle soreness.

Effective Dose: studies support up to 10 grams per day which may be divided into pre and post exercise doses.

Ribose - a naturally occurring sugar made in the body from glucose and an integral component for the production of ATP. In fact, without ribose, ATP cannot be produced. Ribose has been well studied in cardiovascular conditions and shown to improve heart function by increasing levels and availability of ATP in patients with congestive heart failure. Supplementation can increase the heart's oxygen threshold and restore oxygen utilization for energy metabolism. One small study found that ribose lessened muscle soreness and enhanced the ability to overcome fatigue in people suffering from chronic fatigue or fibromyalgia. For athletes, it is interesting to note that studies show a significant reduction in the level of adenosine nucleotide - the structural backbone of ATP - in muscle after strenuous activity. Since ribose is important for the production of adenosine, it is a preferred sugar to support energy production in the cell. Ribose, unlike dietary sugars, has no caloric value since it is not metabolized as fuel.

Effective Dose: studies support 5 g to 10g per day. Use a reputable source of ribose such as from Bioenergy Life Science®.

Carbohydrates – carbohydrates are stored as glycogen in muscles and liver, which can be called upon to provide glucose for ATP production when needed. Dietary restriction of dietary carbohydrates, intense exercise, or endurance training can rapidly deplete glycogen stores. Carbohydrates and glycogen stores in athletes have an important impact on nerve and muscle integration that effects performance. Studies show that when glycogen levels are depleted and dietary carbohydrate intake is restricted, ATP production is hindered and this affects the nerves that activate muscles to do work. Pay particular attention to the carbohydrate requirements and modifications in chapter six.

Magnesium - an essential mineral that activates the enzymes ATP-synthase, which is needed to generate ATP. A deficiency of magnesium reduces the ability of muscles to relax properly and has major implications in energy metabolism and oxygen utilization. In a study of healthy individuals,

low magnesium intake increased the need for oxygen during physical activity and those with low magnesium levels tired more quickly. Other findings confirm that low magnesium levels increase the effort of muscles to work effectively regardless of whether or not the person was a well-trained athlete. Green vegetables and whole grains are rich sources of magnesium. If considering a supplement, look for chelated forms since they are better absorbed. Try to take divided doses throughout the day as higher amounts can cause loose stools.
Effective Dose: studies support 400 mg daily.

Coenzyme Q10 (CoQ10) – CoQ10 is well studied and acknowledged for its antioxidant and cardioprotective benefits. It plays a primary role in mitochondrial energy production. Studies examining CoQ10 and physical exercise have confirmed its effect for lessening fatigue and improving performance. In addition, as an antioxidant, it has been shown to reduce exercise-induced muscle damage. Lastly, measurements of mean power, fatigue indices, autonomic nervous activity, and increased time to exhaustion have all shown to be positively influenced by supplemental CoQ10.
Effective Dose: studies support 100 mg daily.

Quercetin – a naturally occurring flavonoid found in many fruits, vegetables and some grains, quercetin has exhibited several potent effects as an antioxidant and anti-inflammatory agent. Animal studies have identified a new role for quercetin as a compound that enhances performance and increases mitochondrial synthesis. In a study with untrained individuals, just seven days of quercetin intake increased endurance parameters making it a desirable antioxidant nutrient important to athletes.
Effective Dose: studies support 1,000 mg daily.

The Role of Lactic Acid in Fatigue

Adenosine triphosphate stored in muscles only lasts for a few seconds. The cell quickly begins the resynthesis of ATP using creatine until those stores are depleted as well. Again, we are only talking about an additional few seconds where creatine provides energy for muscle contraction. Once these stores are depleted and intense activity continues (70–90% of maximum heart rate), reliance on anaerobic energy production kicks into gear. The breakdown of glucose to provide energy also yields lactic acid and hydrogen ions as a byproduct. As lactic acid floods the muscle, the notable "burn" is felt and has been implicated as a major cause for fatigue. Well, new research and current thinking tells us to look elsewhere since lactic acid is not the sole culprit.

The complexity behind fatigue can be accounted for by numerous factors including exhausted glycogen stores, anaerobic energy production, decreased levels of ATP and creatine phosphate, and lowered pH (acidity). In fact, research shows that lactic acid may be used as fuel for many tissues and plays a critical role in generating energy during exercise. Once the body recovers from intense activity, lactic acid can be converted to a usable substrate for ATP production. The key here is adequate and efficient recovery since poor clearing of lactic acid can play a role in fatigue and cramping. In addition, chronic elevated lactic acid accumulation contributes to a higher acidic environment which plays a greater role contributing to fatigue. Increased acidity in working muscles slows down enzyme activity, inhibits glucose availability for energy production, and irritates nerve endings. Several studies suggest that buffering agents such as beta-alanine and carnosine may improve performance by reducing acid-induced fatigue.

> **Beta-Alanine/Carnosine** – as intense exercise causes an accumulation of lactic acid and hydrogen ions in muscle tissue, a decrease in pH in muscle creates an acidic state. A nutritional component that buffers pH and decreases acidity is carnosine. Carnosine is produced in muscle from the amino acids L-histidine and beta-alanine. Studies have shown that beta-alanine increases intramuscular carnosine content and helps buffer muscle acidity and lower lactic acid accumulation during prolonged exercise. In addition, beta-alanine seems to be more effective at boosting carnosine synthesis than supplementing with carnosine itself. Using beta-alanine to increase carnosine results in muscle fibers operating in an optimal pH range, which helps maximize their ability to work harder during strenuous physical activity. Studies confirm the importance of beta-alanine for improving performance during short bouts of strenuous activity, delaying the onset of lactic acid production, and buffering excess hydrogen ions.
> **Effective Dose: studies support 4 g to 6 g daily.**

Protecting The Battery!

Dysfunctional or damaged mitochondria can translate to poor ATP production. Damaged mitochondria is a hallmark trait of many degenerative conditions ranging from neurological diseases to cancer to aging. Some of the biggest offenders of mitochondrial damage is free radicals – a subject that we have discussed in chapter three. Free radical production increases as we age and mitochondria, in particular, are an easy target since they consume most of the oxygen taken into the cell and produce some of the deadliest free radicals as a byproduct of ATP production. During strenuous activity, the more oxygen you take in and the more ATP you produce, the more free radicals generated. For the athlete this correlates to fatigue, muscle soreness, and decreased performance and recovery. How effective the body deals with free radicals depends on the training protocol, diet and supplement regimen, and adequate rest. If these conditions are met then the mitochondria are better protected against free radicals. If the importance of diet, supplements, training, and rest aren't addressed, then athletic performance will suffer.

Mitochondrial Support – the genetic material (DNA) found in mitochondria is more susceptible to the destructive effects of free radicals than DNA found elsewhere in the cell. The following nutrients are both potent antioxidants and cofactors in ATP production: coenzyme Q10 (CoQ10), alpha lipoic acid, SOD (GliSODin®), acetyl L-carnitine, and glutathione (Setria®)

*Quick Note On Energy Drinks

The effect of caffeine on performance has been well studied. It seems that moderate amounts of 3 – 6 mg per kg body weight supports endurance and performance. Regarding its use in resistance training, the data is not as convincing with studies showing conflicting results. There are textbooks on this subject that go well above and beyond the scope of this book, and I highly recommend you browse the literature on PubMed (www.pubmed.com). Nevertheless, it's important to briefly address the use and abuse of caffeine found in many worthless pre-workout beverages that litter store shelves. Stuffing hoards of stimulants in the body is not the same as supporting energy production in the body. Many of these so-called "energy drinks" are filled with caffeine and caffeine-like compounds. Herbs like guarana and herba mate may sound natural but contain caffeine-like stimulants. After reading several articles describing the ill effects of over consumption of energy drinks (including seizures, heart failure and death), it is apparent that their problems outweigh the benefits for athletes. The ridiculous amounts of caffeine found in some of these products - some over 500 milligrams - serves no benefit and, in fact, taxes the cardiovascular and nervous systems. The enormous amount of sugar, artificial colors and artificial sweeteners found in some products only add to the problems. Remember, being artificially stimulated with these toxic products does not help the body produce cellular energy efficiently and can have the opposite effect with long term use. So, while caffeine in the correct dosages will contribute to performance in endurance sports and may provide you with initial "push energy" for resistance training, be aware of the amount in the product you take and avoid excess levels.

CHAPTER 5
Exercise and Muscle Breakdown

The hundreds of muscles in the body form an intricate network to produce force and cause motion. To do that, muscles turn the chemical energy found in adenosine triphosphate (ATP) into mechanical energy required to lift a weight or simply walk across a room. The stresses exerted on muscles, and their ability to overcome that stress, is called "adaptation" and is the prerequisite for becoming stronger. Muscles are incredibly capable of adapting to stress and both aerobic and anaerobic exercise help build stronger muscles that are progressively more efficient at storing and utilizing energy. Exercise is simply a stress the body responds to by building larger, stronger muscles.

In order for muscles to grow stronger, they must recover. The bundles of intricate fibers that make up muscle are sensitive to the stress placed on them and susceptible to damage when the demand for work exceeds the ability to recover. Research has confirmed that strenuous exercise traumatizes muscles by causing microscopic tears in the fibers themselves. Increases in free radicals and hormonal and immunological changes also occur. The result is a constellation of symptoms felt after strenuous activity referred to as "delayed onset muscle soreness" (DOMS). The leading cause of DOMS is directly related to the trauma exerted by mechanical forces on muscle tissue during strenuous exercise.

The damage to muscle tissue or loss of muscle mass during strenuous exercise (particularly overtraining) is also common in many degenerative diseases. Thus, we have two seemingly disparate populations experiencing similar metabolic outcomes of progressive weight loss and decreased muscle mass. In severe states, this loss can be as high as five percent! Clinicians refer to this as catabolic wasting, cachexia or wasting syndrome. This process is not always caused by inadequate calories, but rather, one that favors catabolism (breaking down) rather than anabolism (building up) no matter how many calories the person consumes. Research has revealed that this breakdown process is the result of both the disease itself and hormonal and immunological changes such as the release of inflammatory cytokines (IL-1, IL-6, TNFα). Sound familiar? These are some of the same inflammatory messengers we see elevated in the athlete after strenuous exercise! Based on my experience working with immune-compromised conditions (e.g., cancer, AIDS), muscle wasting is a nutritional challenge that is equally shared by the athlete and patient. Therefore, we can view the athlete as a patient and use an approach to recovery similar to that used for degenerative or immune-compromised conditions.

Building Muscle and Protein: Don't Fall for the Numbers Game

In order to withstand greater forces during the next resistance training session, muscles adapt by increasing in strength and mass. After the workout, muscle tissue begins to rebuild itself provided it is allowed enough time and nutrients to recover. This is the rebuilding process and recovery is the key. A healthy diet containing good quality protein (amino acids), carbohydrates, and healthy fats aid in building lean muscle mass. The amino acids found in protein not only build muscle, but also regulate muscle activity, supply energy pathway intermediates and help form healthy ligaments, tendons, and bone – just to name a few.

Although protein is important for muscle repair, the ratio between protein and carbohydrates before and following exercise should also be considered. Carbohydrates positively influence muscle growth by sparing proteins so they can be used to build muscle and prevent its breakdown. Several studies demonstrate that exercise-induced muscle damage may be reduced when consuming a combination of protein and carbohydrates after strenuous exercise. Unfortunately, the exact opposite has been touted by certain sports supplement companies. While exercise has a profound effect on protein metabolism, unscrupulous sports nutrition companies would like you to believe that taking excessive amounts of protein is the answer for all the nutritional needs of the athlete. The level of protein in some of these supplements can be as high as 50 grams or more per serving! Less is more when it comes to protein supplementation during recovery. In fact, protein supplementation may not be necessary considering the typical American diet is already high in protein. Low carbohydrate, high protein diets can push those amounts up even more. Pick up any "muscle" magazine, and you are inundated with messages to consume large amounts of protein, preferentially using a proprietary powder formula. The implication is that burgeoning athletes can be as big and strong as the guy in the advertisement (some who are obviously taking steroids). The truth is that high amounts of protein taxes the kidneys and, in the case of animal protein, can be high in saturated fat. Put the muscle magazine down and take a look at legitimate sports nutrition research on the internet – you may want to start by looking at *The Journal of the International Society of Sports Nutrition* website at http://www.jissn.com.

Avoid the protein numbers game when looking for a post-workout recovery beverage. Unless you are on steroids, you don't need 50 g of protein after exercise. Stick with a post-workout product that provides 20 – 30 g of protein primarily from whey – any more than this and you're wasting your money!

It can't be overemphasized that protein is just one aspect of the multiple nutritional needs of athletes. Addressing other concerns, such as oxidative stress, inflammation, fatigue, and immune suppression is equally important. Post-workout products containing 40 to 50 grams or more of protein per serving is unnecessary and can actually contribute to muscle breakdown by acidifying the body (discussed below). In fact, studies show that the body benefits most from protein when supplied in smaller amounts of no more than 20 to 30 grams. Higher amounts of protein do not result in any further increase in muscle building. This makes sense because the body can only process a certain amount of protein in a single serving. Another comparative study looking at intakes of 90 grams of protein versus 30 grams found that they both provided the same benefit. So, it seems that anything over 30g of protein is a waste of money! When protein requirements for the body are met, any excess breaks down and is used for caloric needs or even converted into fat for storage. All of this is done at the expense of the kidneys that are forced to deal with the excess nitrogen from protein. Building muscle involves more than just protein and is very much affected by your total calorie and carbohydrate intake.

This might be hard for some to swallow but restricting carbohydrates can actually negate the benefits of protein and lead to increased muscle breakdown during and after exercise. Dietary carbohydrates spare proteins so they can be used to build and maintain muscles. The most likely mechanism explaining carbohydrates protein-sparing effect is due to insulin secretion, which is thought to prevent muscle breakdown from occurring. So, make sure to consume at least 30 grams or more of carbohydrate with your protein after exercise since this combination maximizes muscle protein synthesis and helps replenish depleted muscle glycogen stores. For the endurance athlete (e.g., long-distance runner or cycler), 60 or more grams of carbohydrates may be more appropriate. The multiple nutritional needs of the athlete go well above and beyond protein and stimulants as covered throughout this book.

Keep Your Diet Alkaline

Ingesting excess protein can acidify the body and in turn, limit its benefits. Metabolic acidosis (the acidification of the cellular environment) is diet dependent and can increase bone and muscle breakdown and susceptibility to illness. The body tries to defend against acidosis by breaking down bone and muscle to help normalize the acid-base (pH) balance. The more acidic the body, the more the body breaks down muscle and bone to maintain balance.

To combat the acidifying effects of dietary protein, increased consumption of alkaline fruits and vegetables is recommended; even the ones you think are acidic like oranges and grapefruits. Studies have examined the relationship between increasing alkalinity and maintaining muscle and the results have been positive. So, don't just focus on protein and starchy carbohydrates. Make sure to include plenty of fruits and vegetables as often as possible (for a more detailed discussion please read the chapter on dietary manipulation). Lastly, be aware of another body alkalizer: calcium. Results of a 12-year follow-up study looking for an association between hip fracture risk and high-protein diets found that high intakes of protein coupled with less than 800 milligrams of calcium daily increased the risk of hip fractures three times more compared to those with a lower protein intake. Make sure to consume sufficient calcium. If you need to supplement, chelated forms, such as calcium citrate, are preferred because of their better absorption.

Sleep: The often Neglected Performance Factor

Unfortunately, while most athletes know rest is important, that doesn't stop them from training constantly. The fact is that rest is critical for muscles to repair and rebuild. Inadequate rest leads to the elevated levels of stress hormones like cortisol. Released from the adrenal glands, cortisol is a catabolic hormone that antagonizes muscle repair. Adequate, deep sleep promotes the release of the anabolic hormones testosterone and growth hormone that aid in the recovery and repair of muscle tissue. Lastly, there is new research suggesting that the muscle itself expresses circadian genes, which control muscle protein synthesis! Hence, pulling an all-nighter could cause dysregulation in these genes, which in turn, negatively affects the muscle building processes. At least 8 hours is absolutely necessary to maintain healthy muscle.

Menacing Cortisol: It's Back!

As discussed in chapter two, rising levels of cortisol is part of the normal physiological response to the stress of exercise. But that response comes at a price: inflammation, muscle breakdown, and altered testosterone levels. When glucose stores in muscle are exhausted, cortisol kicks in, breaking down muscle and fat for conversion to glucose for energy. This process is called "gluconeogenesis" and is necessary when the body needs fuel. Once the stress is removed, cortisol levels quickly normalize. But overtraining and inadequate rest prolongs the cortisol response, favoring catabolism, and decreases anabolic hormones like testosterone. It is important to normalize cortisol levels as quickly as possible while maintaining testosterone levels. Studies have shown that dietary carbohydrates, when added to a protein beverage, blunt rising cortisol and help maintain testosterone levels after strenuous activity. When carbohydrates were restricted, the opposite effect was seen. So, if you are one of the many carbohydrate-phobic individuals, you may be doing more damage than good!

Just Say No To NO Stimulants?

One of the most popular supplements used by young athletes today is nitric oxide (NO) boosters. Typically, a combination of arginine, caffeine and other accessory ingredients, NO boosters are purported to increase blood flow to the muscles by dilating blood vessels – an effect that normally occurs anyway during strenuous exercise without NO boosters. Nitric oxide boosters are a hot topic that athletes have been misled about.

Voted "Molecule of the Year" in Science magazine in 1992, nitric oxide is a very important molecule because it acts as a cellular messenger in numerous biochemical and physiological activities. Some of these include acting as a neurotransmitter in the brain and supporting the immune response. But NO is a dual edge sword that can be detrimental when overly produced in the body. As a matter of fact, chronic elevation of NO is toxic and associated with several disease conditions ranging from cancer to multiple sclerosis. In high levels, it can even act as a free radical. Because excessive levels of NO may be harmful, the body has developed feedback mechanism to actually suppress its production. Nevertheless, the popularity of NO boosters cannot be denied and the benefit of taking these supplements focuses on its ability to dilate blood vessels and increase blood flow to muscles. The critical information often left out of these claims – besides the side effects of taking NO boosters – is the large amounts of the active compound needed to elicit this effect. Arginine, the primary ingredient found in these formulas, is a precursor for manufacturing NO. Studies have demonstrated that intravenous infusions as high as 30 grams stimulate NO production. Oral doses using the same amount are impractical because the large amount of arginine could cause significant side effects and even taking 30 grams in divided doses throughout the day doesn't have a significant effect.In addition to the arginine/NO connection, smaller oral doses of arginine in the five to ten gram range are purported to raise levels of growth hormone, but exercise is a more potent stimulator of growth hormone that arginine alone!

Be aware of the ingredients in the Supplement Facts on the label. It is important that you know how much of each active ingredient you are actually getting on a per serving basis. If you don't see them individually listed, request the information from the company regarding the specific components of the blend.

It is important to understand that arginine is a very important amino acid in sports nutrition that exerts a positive influence on muscle growth and recovery. As an example, new data shows that taking smaller doses (three to ten grams) of arginine can positively affect time to exhaustion and fatigue threshold and improve performance. Most of the claims for arginine are centered on its NO-boosting effect. But that must be taken into context. Many sports supplements formulated to boost NO levels fall grossly short of their claim because they don't meet the required dosage of active compounds (specifically arginine). There are no studies that demonstrate vasodilation effects from the doses commonly found in these types of products on the market. So why are they still so popular? Many sports supplements add high doses of caffeine and caffeine-like components that give the illusion of increased energy, but ultimately are just another high-priced stimulant that does not support energy production in the cell.

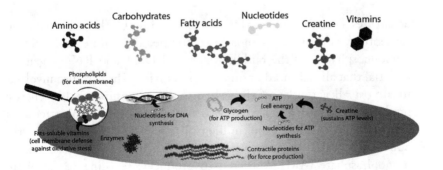

Muscle Driver Supplements: The Primary Players

In addition to the dietary recommendations outlined in chapter six, the primary nutrients that influence muscle growth and maintenance include whey protein, nucleotides, creatine, branched chain amino acids, glutamine, and ribose. More esoteric supplements include ornithine alphaketoglutarate (OKG), hydroxyl methylbutarate (HMB), and citrulline. I recommend the latter supplements be used on a limited basis; cycling their use four weeks on followed by a few weeks off until you achieve your goal. After that, stick with manipulating your diet to supply sufficient calories, good quality protein, complex carbohydrates, and essential fats.

Whey Protein – out of all the protein choices available, whey really outshines them all. From a clinical standpoint, whey not only has the highest biological value (all the essential amino acids in adequate amounts to build muscle), but is the only protein to provide important peptides that support immune function. Whey protein is also rich in the amino acid cysteine, which is needed to build glutathione, an essential antioxidant. In addition, whey is considered a fast acting protein that is able to be digested easier and deliver its amino acids faster compared to other proteins. Lastly, whey is a rich source of branched chain amino acids that can be metabolized into other fuel substrates by muscle tissue. Recent studies confirm whey protein's superiority to other proteins such as soy, and very effective when combined with small amounts of casein. In particular, whey has a greater effect in building muscle at both rest and after exercise. There is also evidence to show that whey protein improves recovery, reduces muscle soreness and breakdown and lowers inflammatory markers such as tumor necrosis factor (TNFα). Look for clean whey protein isolates void of artificial sweeteners and artificial flavors.
Effective Dose: look for whey protein isolates delivering 20 - 30 g per serving. May be combined with a small amount of casein.

Nucleotides - just as amino acids are the building blocks of protein, the nucleotides adenosine, guanosine, cytodine, thymidine and uridine monophosphates are the building blocks of DNA and RNA – genetic material that all cells need to function and divide. They are also involved in almost all activities of the cell including immune health, energy production and muscle tissue synthesis. Muscles recovering from strenuous exercise require millions and millions of nucleotides for tissue growth. Some nucleotides act as cellular messengers, such as cyclic adenosine monophosphate (AMP), or used to produce adenosine triphosphate

(ATP) and adenosine diphosphate (ADP), the chemical energy that drives muscles activity. In clinical settings, nucleotides are critical for repair and recovery from tissue damage, muscle loss and immune suppression. Nucleotides are considered conditionally essential when the demand for them exceeds what the body can produce – especially during periods of rapid growth and repair. So important are nucleotides that they have been used in infant formulas and clinical settings to support post-operative recovery and rehabilitation after injury. In order to maximize growth and repair of muscle and other vital proteins, an adequate supply of nucleotides is necessary. While the data on supplemental nucleotides in athletes concerns itself with immune and hormone response (see chapter two), their functional role during muscle growth warrants serious consideration.

Effective Dose: Studies support 500 - 1500 mg daily.

Creatine – creatine is one of the most popular and controversial supplements on the market. Hundred of studies support creatine's role in increasing muscle strength, mass, and recovery – especially in those with low creatine levels. It plays a critical role in regenerating ATP during strenuous exercise so muscle work can continue. The more ATP generated, the more muscle cells can work. Creatine is especially effective during anaerobic exercises but recent data points to its positive contribution during aerobic exercise as well. Its safety is well established since intermittent use in healthy individuals does not harm the kidneys as some fear. Those with kidney or liver conditions should seek advice from a healthcare professional before using creatine.

As a matter of fact, creatine is gaining recognition outside of sports circles and has several applications in the medical marketplace. Creatine's role in improving muscular strength has now been extended to those with neuromuscular and heart disease. As a neuro-protective agent, creatine is now being studied and used in people suffering from Parkinson's, Huntington's disease, and ALS (amyotrophic lateral sclerosis). New research has focused on the role of creatine in diabetes. When combined with an exercise program, improvements in blood sugar control were shown in type 2 diabetics by increasing glucose transportation into the cell. No negative effects on kidney function were seen. For sports applications, dosing recommendations of creatine initially begin with a "loading phase" of 5 to 20 grams for several days followed by a maintenance dose of two to three grams. However, several studies now demonstrate that the smaller two to three gram dosing for several weeks may be just as effective. So it may be possible to forego the loading phase altogether. Long-term effects and whether it continues to provide muscle enhancement or plateaus at some point still need to be investigated. For this reason and especially if you are considering other players listed below, my recommendation is short term use of 3 to 5 grams daily for four weeks followed by several weeks off – repeat cycling until desired goals are achieved.

Effective Dose: Studies support 3 - 5 g daily that can be split before and after exercise. Until published data shows other forms are superior, creatine monohydrate is the preferred and most studied form.

Branched Chain Amino Acids (BCAAs) – BCAAs are essential amino acids that include leucine, isoleucine, and valine. While popular among sports supplements, BCAAs have a long history of use in clinical settings for illnesses such as amyotrophic lateral sclerosis (also known as Lou Gehrig's disease) and chronic hepatic encephalopathy (a liver disease that affects the brain). Branch chain amino acids have also been used in immuno-compromised conditions such as cancer to help reduce muscle wasting and improve appetite. They are also useful as a nutritional treatment for stress and infections in hospitalized patients. For the athlete, BCAAs are critical for muscle function and growth. They can be used by muscle tissue for energy production. The longer and harder the workout, the more BCAAs are called upon for use as energy in muscle. As we've discussed in chapter four, BCAAs have the ability to combat central fatigue since they compete for tryptophan in the brain, which prevents increased levels of serotonin (a neurotransmitter that may contribute to feeling tired and fatigued). Leucine is the most effective for stimulating muscle growth and preventing breakdown. Studies have confirmed that the administration of several grams of BCAAs before and after strenuous exercise significantly reduce the breakdown of muscle. Other studies have pointed to the effect of BCAAs acting on key enzymes involved in protein synthesis and suppressing exercise-induced muscle degradation in both resistance and endurance activity. It is important to use BCAAs before and after the workout to spare muscle tissue from breaking down and support recovery.

Effective Dose: Studies support 200 mg BCAA's per kg of bodyweight daily– dose may be split before and after exercise.

Glutamine - glutamine is the most abundant free amino acid in the body and is involved in numerous biochemical and biological functions, including maintenance of muscle tissue and immune health. It is particularly important for metabolically active cells including those of the immune system, intestinal tract and muscle as it is stored and used by these tissues during periods of intense physical stress. Glutamine is concentrated in muscle tissue where it can be stored or released during stressful periods. This is why many hospital-based nutritional formulas are supplemented with glutamine and have been used for the nutritional treatment of trauma, infections, burns and post-operative recovery. For the athlete, glutamine can help replenish glycogen stores in muscle and minimize muscle breakdown. Strenuous exercise can significantly deplete glutamine stores and, thus, warrants supplementation. Glutamine is one of the most important nutrients influencing muscle recovery after strenuous exercise.

Effective Dose: Studies support 5 - 10 g daily, which may be split before and after exercise.

Ornithine alpha-ketoglutarate (OKG) - with over two decades of clinical use, OKG limits muscle wasting in several conditions. OKG has been used extensively in clinical settings as part of the nutritional treatment for burn patients, trauma conditions, and malnourished states where it has been shown to decrease the breakdown of muscle while increasing its synthesis. At doses exceeding 12 grams, studies of hospitalized patients suggest that OKG blocks the catabolic effects of cortisone and directly stimulates the release of growth hormone. Also, OKG restores glutamine levels in muscle, which is significantly decreased during strenuous exercise. Several studies have pointed to the unique ability of OKG to stimulate the release of anabolic hormones like insulin and growth hormone. While OKG has not been formerly studied in athletes, its ability to stimulate the release of anabolic hormones and preserve glutamine levels in muscle tissue warrants consideration as a potentially important supplement for the athlete.

Effective Dose: Studies support 10 - 25 g daily.

Hydroxymethyl Butarate (HMB) - HMB is a metabolite of the important BCAA leucine and is produced when muscles break down after strenuous activity. For critical care patients, post-operative or wasting conditions, HMB may improve nitrogen balance and muscle gain. When combined with other amino acids, HMB may reverse the breakdown of lean tissue in immuno-compromised conditions (e.g. cancer, AIDS). With respect to athletes, the data is inconclusive. Studies utilizing three grams daily with resistance exercise have only demonstrated moderate recovery of muscle function after exercise-induced muscle damage and some positive effects during aerobic activity. Larger doses in untrained individuals or elderly subjects have reduced the symptoms associated with exercise-induced muscle damage and increased muscle mass following one year of administration. Thus, it appears that athletes undertaking high volume training (i.e., two-a-days, long distance running, etc.) may benefit the most from this product.

Effective Dose: Studies support 3g daily.

Citrulline - is an amino acid and in the form of citrulline-malate has been shown to improve protein synthesis by acting on the enzymes required for efficient muscle building. Other noted effects include increasing growth hormone and positively affecting arginine availability for nitric oxide synthesis. While a study demonstrated that citrulline might reduce post-exercise muscle soreness and improve performance, it did not have a control group and requires further study. Nevertheless, the multiple positive effects citruilline has initially demonstrated, makes it a very promising nutrient.

Effective Dose: Studies utilized 3g daily.

Putting It All Together

A perfect example of utilizing many of the nutrients described in chapters 2 – 5 can be found in the study entitled "*The effects of a post-workout nutraceutical drink on body composition, performance and hormonal and biochemical responses in Division I college football players*"

Comparative Exercise Physiology, September 2009. The study examined the impact of supplementing the diet of college football players with a recovery drink (Surgex®) containing whey, SOD, CoQ10, ribose, nucleotides, beta glucans and other nutrients. Specific parameters examined included changes in performance, peak power, body composition, anabolic status (testosterone:cortisol), and recovery (oxidative stress & inflammatory markers) during pre-season conditioning. Up against a leading sports nutritional supplement, it was found that this specialized nutraceutical drink provided statistically significant improvements in all parameters and addressed the multiple nutritional needs of athletes above and beyond excess protein and stimulants.

CHAPTER 6
Dietary Manipulation:
Challenges & Health Concerns

Genetics and training have a huge impact on athletic performance. However, you can maximize your potential with proper nutritional strategies including diet manipulation and supplement use. Think of your body as a machine – you have an engine and you supply fuel for that engine to run efficiently. Well, if you do not supply enough fuel or use poor quality fuel, your health and performance is affected. Understanding the strategy of dietary manipulation and nutrient timing are key concepts to achieving energy demands, optimal body composition and peak performance. Unfortunately, it's very common for athletes to have an imbalance of the right type of calories. Dietary manipulation goes beyond calories; it is more about what those calories are made of, when they are consumed and what other types of calories we consume with them. Before we discuss these important concepts, let's take a look at some hurdles that keep an athlete from reaching their nutritional goals.

In modern society, nutrient rich choices are not always easy to come by. With all the marketing and mis-information from the food industry and certain bodybuilding supplement companies, an athlete is often confused by what is "healthy." In addition, many coaches or sports teams do not have access to a board certified, licensed nutritionist or certified sports dietitian to help establish nutrition goals and translate those goals into strategies. This can result in less than optimal health and performance and places the athlete at risk of missing key nutrients, having an imbalance of fuel, and lacking knowledge about supplements and the dangers of fad diets. All it takes is a trip to the grocery store to compare the small amount of whole foods on the shelves and the thousands of processed items vying for your attention. Eating out? Fast food restaurants sit on every corner with "supersize" menu options loaded with saturated fats and sugar. Even the Federal government, which spends only $3.6 million on the "5 A Day Program" (a governmental program promoting the consumption of more fruits and vegetables), can't compete against the food industry's $25 billion spending spree for promoting their products. When is the last time you saw a commercial encouraging you to eat broccoli?

Unfortunately, it is not uncommon to find athletes consuming high amounts of sugar and fat or, conversely, following a low carbohydrate, high protein diet. Our busy lifestyles present challenges to obtaining optimal nutrition. The answer: have a plan (i.e. nutrient timing, nutrient dense foods) and support. The coach is a key player in this process. They have perhaps the strongest influence on athletes' attitudes about nutrition. If the coach doesn't send the message that optimal fuel intake is important, or incorrect information is provided, the athlete is unlikely to listen to anyone else who encourages proper fueling. Coaches have so many responsibilities that proper nutrition often gets overlooked. Turning to an expert such as a qualified registered and certified sports dietitian can be an asset to the whole team.

An evaluation of the diets and eating habits of 345 male and female NCAA athletes showed an inadequate supply and quality of fuel. Only one out of four athletes ate enough calories to fuel their training and competitions. The motivation to either lose weight and/or change body composition seems to result in under-eating for many athletes. The study also showed male athletes were more likely to consume more fat, saturated fat, and cholesterol than female competitors. For these athletes, fat is displacing carbohydrate as an energy source, contributing to their inadequate carbohydrate intake. Take a look at the following athlete's diet that had enough fuel (calories), yet too much sugar and saturated fats. By exchanging the types of carbohydrates and fats in his diet (dietary manipulation) for more complex carbohydrates (e.g. fruit, vegetables, whole grains) and more unsaturated fats (e.g. fish, nuts, avocado) the body will respond metabolically different.

Male Football Athlete, Running Back, Weight: 250 lb. (114 kg)

Breakfast: . . . . 20 oz bottle Gatorade, 6 mini doughnuts, chocolate frosted
Lunch: . . . . 1 Big Mac, 1 large order french fries, 32 oz Coke, 1 large chocolate shake
Dinner: . . . . 1-12 inch supreme pizza, thin crust, 6 breadsticks with cheese sauce and 32 oz Coke

Nutrient	Actual Intake	Recommended Intake
Energy (kcal)	6,235	5,000
Carbohydrate (g)	824	684-1140
Protein (g)	161	180
Fat (g)	260	55-165
Saturated fat (g)	80	<33

Adapted and modified from Hinton PS et al. Int J Sport Nutr Exerc Metab. 2004 Aug;14(4):389-405. Nutrient intakes and dietary behaviors of male and female collegiate athletes.

Another study found NCAA Division I women's soccer players failed to meet carbohydrate intake to promote refueling of muscles and missed the minimum needs of several vitamins and minerals (e.g. folate, copper, magnesium and vitamin E) even though they seemed to have met total caloric needs during training. Studies have found that female cross-country runners met only 50 percent of their calcium needs in their diet - an average intake of 605 milligrams per day – compared to the recommended amount of 1,000-1,200 milligrams per day. Lastly, the diets of 72 elite female athletes from a variety of sports failed to meet the requirements for folate, calcium, magnesium, and iron.

Let's look at the health of 70 NCAA football linemen, average age 20 years old, that were evaluated for abdominal obesity, blood pressure, blood glucose, cholesterol, triglycerides, upper-body skinfolds, and waist circumference. All these factors increase the risk for cardiovascular disease and diabetes; a condition known as "metabolic syndrome." Of the 70 athletes, 34 were found to have metabolic syndrome. Just because these athletes are young and active and meet their calorice needs does not mean they are protected from cardiovascular disease and other health issues. In other words, the quality of calories may be more important that the quantity.

This leads to over fueling with poor calorie sources. Instead of acquiring nutrients from food, a dependency on supplements results. Ultimately, fuel sources and nutrient balance is impaired. Energy bars and protein drinks can have a place in an athlete's diet and when whole foods are not available or tolerated, they work great. However, it has been shown some athletes lack knowledge on their use and purpose. A study of 31 freshman NCAA football players showed over 50 percent believed that while adequate protein intake from diet and supplements is necessary for muscle growth and development, protein was the primary source of energy for muscle, and vitamin and mineral supplements increased energy levels. Nothing could be further from the truth!

Dietary Manipulation: All Calories Are Not Alike

The usable energy from food is measured as a calorie and athletes need to be aware that not all calories are the same. There are three nutrients that give us energy from the foods and drinks we consume: carbohydrates and protein provide four calories per gram and fat provides nine calories per gram. Defining energy balance by this concept seems simple; a calorie is a calorie no matter where it comes from. If you eat 10 grams of carbohydrates (10 grams x 4 calories) and 10 grams of protein (10 grams x 4 calories) they both offer 40 calories of fuel. But the body processes and metabolizes carbohydrates, protein and fat very differently. When we eat, the body uses a range of energy to digest, absorb, and metabolize the food we eat. This is known as the thermic (heat) effect of feeding. The body actually burns calories to process the food or drink we consume. The energy cost to digest fat is 2% to 3%, carbohydrate is 6% to 8% and protein 25% to 30%. In other words, the more calories it costs to breakdown food, the more calories are burned or lost as heat (i.e. not stored in the body). Eating 100 calories of fat provides 97-98 calories, 100 calories of carbohydrate provides 92-94 calories, and 100 calories of protein provides 70-75 calories.

The second way to differentiate between calories is to determine the quality of those calories. For example, one cup of baby spinach has 20 times more vitamins A, five times more vitamin C, and three times more calcium than a calorically equivalent amount of iceberg lettuce. This doesn't include all the antioxidants and flavonoids spinach has to offer, such as beta-carotene and lutein. Another example is using fresh avocado to spread on a turkey sandwich instead of mayonnaise; you get more nutrients, fiber and healthy fats in the avocado. Calories from whole foods provide more antioxidants, omega 3 fatty acids, fiber, probiotics, vitamins and minerals than calories from processed foods. If you want to boost energy, support immune system, reduce inflammation and be lean, eat whole, unprocessed foods. Calorie for calorie they are far superior.

Foods that pack in a lot of nutrients per calorie are known as "nutrient-dense foods." Sweets and soft drinks are very low in nutrient density, while fruits, vegetables, fish, whole grains, low fat dairy and lean protein are nutrient dense. See chart below for a list of nutrient dense foods to promote performance and health.

Peak Performance Foods

Fruits: Blueberries, cherries, raspberries, plums, pears, kiwis, mangoes, pineapple, papaya, citrus, bananas, tart cherries, acai, grapes, strawberries, pomegranate, apples, dried fruits, melon, peaches

Vegetables: broccoli, carrots, kale, tomatoes, bell peppers, spinach, sweet potatoes, onions, sun-dried mushrooms, collard greens, arugula, bitter broccoli
Whole Grains: brown rice, pasta, breads, steel cut oats, cereals, quinoa, popcorn, bran, barley
Lean Protein: beans, fish, free-range chicken, grass-fed beef (round or loin cuts), skinless turkey & chicken, pork tenderloin, wild game, whey protein powder
Low Fat Dairy: Greek yogurt, cottage cheese, milk, milk substitutes (oat, rice & almond milk)
Healthy Fats: olive oil, nuts, seeds, avocado, peanut butter, ground flaxseed, salmon, tuna, herring, mackerel, canola oil, eggs (fortified with EPA/DHA), dark chocolate
Spices/Antioxidants: turmeric (curcumin), cinnamon, ginger, garlic, oregano, basil, tea

Why should the athlete, who is metabolically active, be concerned about calories coming from sweets and fatty foods? Sugary and fried foods trigger an inflammatory response in the body. The high intake of refined sugar and low intake of fiber, contribute to abrupt fluctuations in insulin and blood sugar. In the absence of activity, high amounts of sugar stimulate fat production with the eventual outcome being a "sugar crash." Alternatively, energizing the body with 1 cup of Greek yogurt, 1/3 cup blueberries and eight ounces of water provide calories for energy as well as nutrients without the same effect on blood sugar as eating sweets would have.

Another inflammatory booster is the lack of healthy fats due to the food industry offering hefty doses of omega 6 fatty acids (pro-inflammatory) which compete with omega 3 fatty acids (anti-inflammatory). The body metabolizes omega 3 differently than omega 6 and studies have shown less inflammation, improved mood and better body composition with higher intakes of omega 3 fatty acids.

Poor Performance Foods
Sweets/Baked Goods: soda, candy, pastries, cake, cookies, table sugar, syrups
Fatty/Fried Foods: French fries, potato chips, donuts, gravies, cream sauces, fast food burgers
Refined Grains: white bread, bagels, white rice, pasta, cereals

Nutrient Timing

Just like training, nutrition needs to be adapted to the sport, season, and goals. Adapting nutrition periodization into training periodization (according to season or yearly cycles) can provide positive performance changes in energy level, body composition, recovery and reduce the risk of injury. For example, at specific times of the sporting season, one may need more or less carbohydrates to optimize the training and performance. Therefore, athletes need to manage carbohydrates, protein, and fat separately to achieve optimal body size, body composition and maximize performance. Athletes wanting to get leaner would be advised to eat high quality carbohydrates with high fiber content and lean protein sources. Protein is known to reduce appetite and offer more satiety per calorie than carbohydrate and fat and the proportion of carbohydrate, protein, and fat has a significant effect on body composition and weight loss. A study at the University of Washington showed a group of 19 subjects following a 15% protein diet versus a 30% diet. The higher protein diet resulted in 441 calories less per day and average loss of eight pounds of fat over 10 weeks. A similar study also showed a loss of more fat weight following a higher protein diet (34% protein, 46% carbohydrate, 20% fat) versus higher carbohydrate diet (17% protein, 64% carbohydrate, 20% fat).

The timing of calories, the number of meals per day and the size of the meal also influence how the body will respond to calories. In the morning when energy levels are low, breakfast calories are more likely to be used for energy or stored as glycogen (stored carbohydrates) or used to make muscle proteins after an overnight fast versus storing them as fat. After exercising, the body soaks up calories for energy and uses them for muscle repair and building. Given the same number of calories over the course of the day, studies have shown athletes build more muscle and gain less body fat if some of those total calories are consumed within two hours of exercise.

In studies with athletes, meal frequency as a dietary manipulation strategy has also shown to have an effect on body composition. In one particular case, while the amounts of calories were exactly the same, boxers eating six meals per day lowered their body fat percent significantly more than boxers eating two meals per day. Distributing calories evenly throughout the day helps the body stay leaner and keeps blood sugar stable. Ideally, one should be eating every two to three hours as small frequent feedings are burned and utilized by the body more efficiently than gorging fewer larger meals. The first step to optimize individual training and performance through nutrition is to ensure the athlete is consuming adequate calories to balance energy expenditure or meet needs of weight management (gain/loss). We will then look at each nutrient in more detail, along with fueling guidelines for the strength athlete and endurance athlete.

Total calories

To calculate body weight into kilograms: weight in pounds ÷ 2.2 = kilograms (kg)

Training/Goal	Duration	Frequency	Energy IN
General Fitness	30-45 min	3x/week	25-35 Kcal/kg/day
Light-Moderate	45-60 min	3-4x/week	35-40 Kcal/kg/day
Moderate	1-3 hr intense	5-6x/week	40-55 Kcal/kg/day
	3-6 hr high volume	1-2x/week in 5-6 day week	
Heavy/ Competition	2-4 hr	Intense, twice daily	50-80 Kcal/kg/day
Weight Loss	x	x	Subtract 300-500 Kcal/day (food or exercise)
Weight Gain	x	x	Add 300-500 Kcal/day (food)

Adapted and Modified from Leutholtz B, Kreider R: Exercise and Sport Nutrition. **In *Nutritional Health*. Edited by: Wilson T, Temple N. Totowa, NJ: Humana Press; 2001:207-39. 19**

Dietary Manipulation: Carbohydrates

Athletes and coaches are probably more confused about carbohydrates than any other nutrient. Carbohydrates are divided into two main categories: simple (sugars) and complex (starches, fiber). The main difference is the number of glucose links each carbohydrate contains: the more links, the more complex. Common simple sugars include glucose, fructose, sucrose, and lactose. These are found in honey, fruit, juice, milk, table sugar, soda, candy, and included in processed foods using high-fructose corn syrup. Complex carbohydrates include starches such as grains, legumes, vegetables, breads, pasta, rice, cereals, and potatoes.

According to the USDA, in the past seven years, sugar consumption has increased by nearly 20 percent, mainly as high-fructose corn syrup. The USDA recommends limiting added sugars to 40 grams (10 teaspoons) for a 2,000-calorie diet. One 12-ounce soda easily meets this recommendation. The amount of sugar is even more in common soda sizes of 20 and 32-ounces (a 32-ounce soda contains about 91 grams of sugar). The amount of sugar rich, nutrient poor beverages has escalated in the past two decades and is associated with increased body fat and diabetes. As far as the USDA recommendatios go, most nutritionists disagree and prefer to lower simple sugars significantly as part of the diet.

More complex carbohydrates as found in whole grains, fruits, and vegetables help stabilize blood sugars between trainings. If needed, faster digesting carbohydrates like sports drinks, juice, and gels are better taken before, during, and immediately after training only and not to be part of the daily dietary meal intake. During digestion carbohydrates break down into the simple sugars with glucose being the primary fuel. With sufficient intake, the body stores unused glucose in the muscles and liver as an energy reserve (glycogen) for the body to do work. We typically have about 1500-2000 calories of fuel from glycogen storage to use for energy. To put that into perspective for an endurance athlete, one could last about 20 miles before the fuel light comes on. It would vary for a strength and power athlete since high intense workouts rely on carbohydrates as the primary fuel. Essentially, carbohydrates can help build muscle, limit break down of muscle tissue, provide energy for intense training, and enhance recovery for the next training session. Low carbohydrate intakes (i.e. low carb diets) are known to impair athletic performance, suppress immune system and decrease mental function. If glycogen stores are low, the athlete's ability to perform and recover is impaired.

It is more accurate to determine guidelines in relation to carbohydrate grams, rather than energy percentage. Keep in mind, sports nutrition is a combination of art and science when it comes to individualizing caloric and nutrient requirements for each individual. Dietary manipulation involves varying carbohydrates, protein and fat intake according to training demands. Adjusting needs can occur daily and during different cycles or periods of the training phases. For example, an Olympic triathlete's base period (i.e. low to moderate aerobic activity) of training requires an estimated 3 - 5 g/kg/day of carbohydrates. As intensity and duration increases so does the amount of carbohydrate requirements - up to 7 to 10 g/kg/day during competition period.

Estimate Daily Carbohydrate Needs

Endurance Athletes & Intermittent Team Sports

Training	Carbohydrate Intake Target (Daily)
General fitness: less than 1 hr, light to moderate intensity Metabolic Efficiency (periodization: aerobic training/base cycle, weight loss)	3-5 g/kg
Less than 1 hr of moderate intensity exercise, or many hours of predominantly low intensity exercise	5-7 g/kg
More than 1 to 4 hr of moderate to heavy exercise	7-10 g/kg
4 or more hours of moderate intensity exercise, high volume and intense exercise. (Ultraendurance Ironman, Tour de France cyclists)	10-12+ g/kg

Adapted and Modified from L.Burke and E. Coyle, 2004, Nutrition for Athletes," Journal of Sports Sciences 22(1):39-55.

Strength/Power Athletes

Training	Carbohydrate Target (Daily)
Less than 1 hr of light-moderate, weight loss/cutting exercise	2-4 g/kg/day
1 to 2 hr moderate exercise	5-7 g/kg/day
Spring training/two-a-days/heavy	8-10 g/kg/day

Dietary Manipulation: Protein

Manipulating protein in the diet depends on the intensity of exercise, body composition goals and nutrient timing. Just like calories, not all proteins are equal. Protein sources differ in amino acid profile, rate of digestion and/ or absorption, fat provided and metabolic activity. Whey, casein, and soy are digested at different rates, which directly affects whole body breakdown (catabolism) and building (anabolism). Whey is a fast absorbing protein while soy and casein are medium and slow absorbing, respectively. Whey is rich in branched chain amino acids (leucine, isoleucine and valine), immune enhancing ingredients, like immunoglobins and lactoferrin, and proven to stimulate protein synthesis during muscle recovery. Casein, the primary protein in milk, helps to minimize the breakdown of muscle tissue, but is more difficult to digest and is slower acting. Practical application includes the use of 10g whey protein before exercise and 20 – 30g after exercise for immediate availability. On the other hand, application of the slower digested casein (10 - 20 g) provides benefits over a longer time period, such as taking at night before bed. Protein drinks are easy and convenient, yet benefits are also seen when using protein from whole foods as well. The best whole food sources of low fat, high quality protein are skinless chicken, fish, egg whites, Greek yogurt and skim milk (casein and whey). Excellent vegetarian sources include beans, nuts, seeds, quinoa, and soy protein.

Protein should be taken in divided doses of no more than 20 to 40 grams per feeding and be taken with carbohydrates for optimal benefits. Smaller doses offered frequently give the body a continuous flow of amino acids to support energy production (although minimal), tissue growth, enzyme production, hormone synthesis, antibody defenses, fluid and electrolyte balance, and acid-base balance. Ingesting protein beyond what is necessary to meet protein needs does not promote additional gains in strength and muscle mass.

Endurance Athletes & Intermittent Team Sports

Training	Protein Target (daily)
General Fitness	0.8 -1.0 g/kg
Moderate intensity, High volume, lean tissue maintenance	1.0 – 1.6 g/kg
Teens, new athletes, muscle growth/building, calorie restriction/weight loss	1.4 – 2.0 g/kg
Intermittent high intensity (soccer, basketball, hockey)	1.4 - 1.7 g/kg

Strength/Power

Training	Protein Target (daily)
Moderate Intensity, Lean Tissue Maintenance	1.0 – 1.6 g/kg
High Intensity, High Volume, Weight Loss/Cutting	1.6 - 2.0 g/kg
Teens, New Athletes, Muscle Growth/Building, Calorie Restriction/Weight loss	1.6 – 2.0 g/kg

Adapted and modified from International Society of Sports Nutrition position stand: protein and exercise Journal of the International Society of Sports Nutrition 2007, 4:8 Campbell B, et al.

Dietary Manipulation: Fat

Fat is a very misunderstood yet important nutrient and fuel for athletes. Knowing how much and what type of fat to consume will have an impact on health and performance. The dietary recommendation of total fat intake (based on calories) for athletes is similar to or slightly greater than those recommended for non-athletes. Studies have shown that a low-fat, high-carbohydrate diet (i.e. 15% fat, 65% carbohydrates, 20% protein of total calories), typically eaten by athletes, increases inflammation and decreases anti-inflammatory immune factors, depresses antioxidants, and negatively affects blood lipoprotein ratios. Higher-fat diets appear to maintain circulating testosterone concentrations more than low-fat diets. However, this is not a ticket to eat fried foods, greasy pizza, donuts and potato chips. Even though saturated and unsaturated fats contain the same caloric value of nine calories per gram, the majority of fat in the diet should come from unsaturated fats, along with adequate intake of omega-3 essential fatty acids.

Dietary manipulation of fats includes limiting saturated and trans fats that are typically found in fried and processed foods, fast foods, desserts and baked goods, butter, bacon, sausage, margarine, and refined vegetable oils (corn, safflower, and soybean) while attempting to increase unsaturated fats. Since there are no labeling regulations for fast food, many fast food items can contain high levels of trans fatty acids that may go unnoticed. Creative marketing diverts the focus by using clever statements like "cholesterol-free" and "cooked in vegetable oil." No matter how it's stated, a large serving of French fries contains 6.8 grams of trans fats – a very unhealthy, inflammatory fat!

Saturated fats, trans fats (e.g. arachidonic acid found in animal products) and omega-6 fatty acids are pro-inflammatory and hinder muscle recovery. Over time, chronic inflammation decreases blood flow, which lessens nutrient delivery and waste removal from the muscles. Omega-3 fatty acids have the opposite effect: reducing inflammation and competing against pro-inflammatory compounds. Unfortunately, most people do not consume enough foods high in omega-3 fats. The most biologically active omega-3 compounds are EPA (eicosapentaenoic acid) and DHA (docosahexenoic acid) found in fatty fish (salmon, mackerel, albacore tuna) and algae (plant source).

Data on the benefits of omega-3 fats for athletes has been mixed, possibly due to different doses and different types of athletes. Researchers found that inflammatory markers in the blood decrease with omega-3 fish oil supplementation even though it was not shown to increase performance benefit found with moderate duration (60 minute) aerobic exercise. Nevertheless, the fact that omega-3's can lower inflammation is very important in the overall health and recovery for the athlete. Another possible benefit of omega-3 fatty acids is enhanced lung function in athletes. Research has shown that 3 weeks of fish oil supplementation, rich in EPA and DHA, reduces airway narrowing, airway inflammation, and bronchodilator use in elite athletes and asthmatic individuals with exercise-induced bronchoconstriction (EIB).

Lastly, many fat soluble vitamins (i.e., A, D, E) as well as phytonutrients such as polyphenols and carotenoids act as nature's antioxidants by protecting you from free radicals. To optimally absorb these nutrients you need fat with the meal, for example adding nuts, eggs, avocado, olive oil and/or low fat cheese to your salad can be very beneficial. With the right amount of essential fat at each meal, fat soluble nutrients are better absorbed. It's a team effort.

Endurance

Training	Fat Target (daily)
Weight loss, decrease body fat	0.5 - 1.0 g/kg
Off season, base/aerobic cycle, General Fitness, less than 1 hr light-moderate intensity	0.8 -1.0 g/kg
Race/competition cycle, between 1 to 4 hr moderate to heavy exercise 4 or more hours of moderate intensity exercise, high volume and intense exercise. (Ultraendurance Ironman, Tour de France cyclists)	0.8 - 2.0 g/kg

Strength

Training	Fat Target (daily)
Less than 1 hr training, weight loss/decrease body fat regimen	0.5-1.0 g/kg
1 to 2 hr Moderate Intensity	0.8 – 1.0 g/kg
Spring Training/Two-A-Days/Heavy	0.8 – 1.5 g/kg

Dietary Manipulation: Vitamins & Minerals

According to USDA data, people who eat diets high in sugar get less calcium, fiber, folate, vitamin A, vitamin C, vitamin E, zinc, magnesium, iron, and other nutrients. Only one third of individuals meet the recommended amount for calcium and vitamin D. Only one half of individuals had adequate intakes of magnesium. Some would argue the food today is nutrient poor due to processing, depleted soil, too many hormones, and preservatives. This is particularly true of processed foods. On the other hand, whole fresh foods offer numerous nutrients and a synergy between those nutrients that science is still trying to unravel.

A rule of thumb for a healthy diet is to focus on consuming colorful fruits and vegetables to complement your lean protein, complex carbohydrates and essential fats. Focusing on increased intakes of fruits and vegetables has various health benefits for the athlete because it provides an abundant supply of nutrients, promotes weight loss and possibly improves body composition. The phytochemicals from fruits and vegetables have antioxidant and anti-inflammatory effects that have an important role in recovery. For example, quercetin is a powerful antioxidant and anti-inflammatory compound that can be found in berries, broccoli, apples, onions, and tea. Some studies have shown beneficial effects on performance and boosting immune function when consuming quercetin. Additionally, fruit and vegetables are known to have high levels of salicylates, which is the active anti-inflammatory ingredient in aspirin. Getting more calcium and magnesium from vegetables plays a critical role in bone health, muscle contraction, and may help manage body composition more efficiently. When complemented with high vitamin C fruits, increased iron intake from certain vegetables can address athletes who are prone to iron deficiencies and/or anemia and studies have shown improvement in exercise capacity with adequate iron intake. These are just a few examples of the benefits of increased fruit and vegetable intake as this topic warrants an entire book to fully cover all the details.

Dietary Manipulation: Exception to the rule, "Food First"

Certain conditions, lifestyles or dietary practices could contribute to nutrient deficiencies. For example, vegetarians and people suffering from food allergies or food intolerances could be lacking vitamin D, calcium, iron, vitamin B12, zinc, and omega-3 fatty acids. In particular, vitamin D is perhaps one of the most important nutrients when it comes to optimal health and peak performance. Vitamin D can "switch on" cells to help control our immune system, muscle function, inflammatory responses and mental state. Recent evidence based on blood levels suggests it is extremely difficult to get enough from food sources. Approximately 90 percent of our vitamin D comes from the sun. Sun block creams, avoidance of sunlight and seasonal changes in sun exposure reduce the body's ability to produce sufficient levels of vitamin D. The majority of the U.S. population comes up short on vitamin D due to the inadequate levels that have been recommended for many decades and that includes athletes as well. Numerous studies correlate low vitamin D levels with increased risk of stress fractures, colds/influenza, musculoskeletal pain, depressed mood, inflammation, inadequate immune function and impaired muscle strength.

Bottom Line: Get your 25-hydroxy D blood levels tested. Start supplementing with 1,000-2,000 IU/day of vitamin D3 and adjust according to lab results. Optimal blood level: 50 -75 ng/mL. Take with a meal (vitamin D is best absorbed with some fat) and no need to divide the dose.

Dietary Manipulation: Nutrient Timing & Strategies

What you eat before and after training sessions often determines the speed of recovery and ability to build muscle. Experiments trying to determine the best time to eat and drink for optimal performance have concluded that there is wide variation among individuals. Adaptation to exercise includes many beneficial physiological effects however many athletes are not adherent to recommendations that will optimize their performance and recovery.

Before

Research indicates it is best to consume a small carbohydrate and high quality protein snack 30-60 minutes before an intense bout of exercise. An ideal pre-exercise snack should be low in fat and fiber to ensure that it is easily digested. It should provide sufficient carbohydrates to optimize glycogen levels and satiate hunger.

Endurance & Strength Athletes

Pre-Training	Carbohydrates	Protein
1 hour	1 g/kg	10-20 g
2 hours	2 g/kg	20-40 g
3 hours	3 g/kg	20-40 g
4 hours	4 g/kg	20-40 g

During

Intake of fluids or solids during training depends on many factors: initial fuel levels, duration, intensity, sport, and environment. If training lasts more than one hour, athletes should consume a sports drink to maintain blood glucose levels, help prevent dehydration, and reduce the immunosuppressive effects of intense exercise. The body can burn one gram of carbohydrate per minute or about 60 grams per hour. It has also been shown that combining multiple carbohydrates (e.g., glucose, maltodextrin, sucrose) results in improved availability due to different pathways for each carbohydrate. Moderate to high intensity exercise that lasts between 60 to 90 minutes will deplete glycogen levels. In addition, carbohydrate requirements for exercise are increased in the heat and cold, due to a shift in fuel use towards carbohydrate oxidation. This makes it important to deliver the right nutrients at the right time in order to offset a drop in energy levels. A combination of electrolytes with four to eight percent carbohydrates (e.g., simple sugars, maltodextrin) is ideal for optimal absorption and tissue delivery. More on fluids and hydration will be covered in chapter seven.

During	Carbohydrates	Protein
Light - Max intensity < 45 min	none	none
Moderate - Max intensity 45-60 min	< 30 g	none
Moderate > 1-2 hr	30-60 g	Optional (5-10 g)
Endurance, Submax intensity > 2 hr	30-90 g	Optional (5-10 g)
Team Sports ~90 min), intermittent high intensity	30-60 g	Optional (5-10 gm)

Post-Training (Recovery)
Recovery nutrition starts before a training session even begins. Sounds odd, but if you start a training session low on fuel it will take you longer to recover – especially replensing glycogen and repairing damaged muscle.

Carbohydrates, protein, fluids and electrolytes are crucial post-workout nutrients. The optimal method of replenishing glycogen levels after exercise is to combine a simple sugar with a fast digesting protein (e.g., whey isolate). Implementing this dietary strategy after exercise has been shown to influence protein synthesis, resulting in greater lean mass growth for power athletes.

The combination of these two nutrients causes a sharp rise in insulin, which drives glucose and protein into the muscle cell more efficiently. The recovery process immediately enhances training adaptation and hinders cortisol levels from breaking down muscle tissue further. It speeds up the recovery process by helping the body adapt more efficiently and undo some of the damage (i.e., oxidative stress, immune suppression, muscle damage, fatigue) that is inevitable after strenuous exercise.

Research on immune function in runners shows that carbohydrate supplementation during (approximately 45 g/hr) and immediately after (approximately 45 g) intense prolonged exercise, helped reduce cortisol levels and maintain lymphocyte production, thus preventing infection. Research has shown that post recovery nutrition increases strength, improves body fat percentage with regular strength training and maximizes glycogen replenishment. The ideal ratio of carbohydrates to protein to enhance glycogen loading is 3:1. Glycogen levels can be reloaded slowly, without any negative effect on performance, if more than 24 hours elapse between training sessions. However, if less than 24 hours pass or there are multiple training sessions in a day, then it is highly recommended to reload glycogen stores immediately.

Post-Training	Carbohydrates	Protein
Moderate intensity less than 1 hr	Optional, eat regular meal within 2 hr	Optional, eat regular meal within 2 hr
Next session less than 8 hr, High intensity, high volume	1 – 1.5 g/kg+ within 30-60 min repeat every 2 hr until regular meal	0.25 - 0.50 g/kg or 10-25 g

Adapted from Hawley, J.A. and Burke, L.M. (1998). Peak Performance: Training and Nutritional Strategies for Sport. Sydney: Allen and Unwin.[47] **Kreider RB: Dietary supplements and the promotion of muscle growth with resistance exercise.** *Sports Med* **1999 , 27(2):97-110.**

Carbohydrate Loading

For endurance athletes competing more than 90 to 120 minutes, it is advised to supersaturate glycogen stores two to three days prior to competition. Athletes should taper training by 30 - 50 % and consume 200 to 300 g/day of extra carbohydrates. Several studies suggest that there is a "carbohydrate loading threshold" of 8 to 10 g/kg that is necessary to achieve the performance benefits of carbohydrate loading. Ideally, this strategy should be practiced to see what works best for each individual as studies do show it can improve endurance exercise capacity.

Sample Menu: **Endurance Athlete (e.g., runner, triathlete, cyclist, cross country skier).**

Female, 60 kg (132 lb), moderate intensity

Goal: Lean/5 lb weight loss

Outdoor temperature: 70 degrees, 20% humidity

40-45 Kcal/kg, 6 g/kg carbohydrates, 1.8 g/kg protein, 1.0 g/kg fat

6:30 a.m.: 1 c. steel cut oats mixed with 1 Tbsp. peanut butter & 1 medium banana & 4 oz skim milk, 1 c. water

9:30 a.m.: 6 oz Greek Vanilla Yogurt, 1/2 tsp. cinnamon, 2 Tbsp. oz sliced almonds, 1 c. water

12:30 p.m.: 1 c. minestrone soup, 4 whole grain salted crackers, Salad: 1.5 c. raw spinach leaves, 2 Tbsp. nuts, ½ c. fresh sliced strawberries, 4 oz grilled chicken breast, 2 Tbsp. balsamic vinaigrette dressing

3:30 p.m.: Pre-training (1 to 1.5 hr before a run): ½ of a turkey and low fat cheese sandwich, 10g whey protein drink

4:45 p.m.: Pre-training (15 minutes before) 1 gel packet

5:00 p.m.: During Training (2 hour session)

> **1st hour:** 16 oz water

> **2nd hour:** 16 oz water, 1 gel packet (25 gm carbohydrates - maltodextrin, sucrose)

7:00 -7:30 p.m.: Post-exercise: ½ whole grain bagel, 8 oz smoothie (tart cherry juice, 1 scoop whey protein powder, ½ vanilla yogurt, ice)

8:30 p.m.: 3 oz baked salmon with mango sauce, 1 c. pasta salad, 1 small sweet potato (with 1 tsp. honey and 1 tsp. salted butter), 1 c. steamed broccoli, 1 c. skim milk, 1 c. water

Totals: 2400-2500 Kcal, 375 g carbohydrates, 110 g protein, 60 g fat. 1800 -1900 mg sodium, 35-40 g fiber, 60% carb, 18% protein, 22% fat

<u>**Sample Menu:**</u> **Strength/Power Athlete (e.g., football, hockey, basketball, baseball).**

Male, pro-wide receiver, 90 kg (200 lb), moderate-heavy intensity

Goal: Get leaner

Outdoor Temperature: 80 degrees, 80% humidity

45-50 Kcal/kg, 7 g/kg carbohydrates, 1.8-2.0 g/kg protein, 1.0 g/kg fat

7:30 a.m.: 2 whole grain waffles, 2 Tbsp. real maple syrup, 2 tsp. salted Smart Balance butter, with 1 c. blueberries on top, Omelet: 1 egg, 2 egg whites, 1 c. chopped spinach, 1 Tbsp olive oil, ¼ c. low fat cheese and 1 c. unsweetened iced tea.

10:30 a.m.: 1/3 c. fruit & nut trail mix, 1 Greek yogurt, 1 bag apple slices, 1 c. water

12:30 p.m.: Pre-Training: 16 oz low fat 1% Milk, 1 natural peanut butter and jelly sandwich

2:00 p.m.: During Training (2 hour session: 30 minutes aerobic/indoor stationary bike, 1 hour 30 minutes football (high intensity - speed drills/ plyometrics)

> 1st hour: 20 oz sports drink, 1 c water
>
> 2nd hour: 20 oz sports drink + 1 electrolyte packet (300 mg sodium), 1 c. water

4:00-4:30 p.m.: Post-exercise: 20 – 30g whey protein, 1 fruit/nut bar

6:00 p.m.: 4 oz roasted chicken breast, 1.5 c. cooked brown rice, 1 c. steamed baby carrots, 2 whole grain rolls, 2 c. melon, 8 oz orange juice

9:30 p.m.: 1 c. Greek yogurt, 1 tsp. honey, 1 c. berries, 1.5 c. dry cereal

Totals: 4000-4200 Kcal, 630 g carbohydrates, 175 g protein, 98 g fat. 3200 mg sodium, 40 g fiber, 60% carb, 18% protein, 22% fat

CHAPTER 7
Hydration: Water & Electrolytes – The Underrated Nutrients

Water, water, everywhere, but what is an athlete to drink? There are so many drink choices on the market today that it becomes confusing as to what actually can enhance performance, or at least not hinder it. Many athletes overlook the importance of hydration and ignore the factors that play a part in optimal hydration, including sweat rate, environment, training intensity and duration, age, body size, and even body composition. This chapter deals with the importance of fluid balance and how to monitor your hydration status. Developing a customized fluid and electrolyte plan will also be covered.

Water is a simple molecule composed of two hydrogens and one oxygen atom (H_2O) and provides no direct energy (calories). Yet, it is the most important nutrient for life. Water plays a vital role regulating blood volume and body temperature as well as affecting heart, nerve and muscle function. Energy systems in the body depend on it for optimal function. It provides the medium to transport nutrients across tissues and carry away toxins. It is the base for all biochemical reactions in the body.

Water is stored in two main compartments: inside the cell (called "intracellular") and outside the cell (called "extracellular"). Extracellular spaces include water in the vascular system (i.e. blood and blood plasma), spinal fluids, digestive juices, and miscellaneous sites (e.g. fluid found in the eyes and ears). Total body water for an average adult male is about 60% of body weight and for an average adult female, 50%. Instead of percentages, let's talk volume: approximately 42 liters (11 gallons) for the adult male and 30 liters (8 gallons) for the adult female. Even though the body is primarily composed of water, amounts found between the intracellular and extracellular compartments are not equal in volume. For example, 28 liters is located inside the cells, whereas the remaining 14 liters is outside the cells (i.e. blood). Water moves between these compartments quite easily, allowing for regulation of body temperature, transport of nutrients, removal of wastes, and acting as a medium for biochemical reactions occurring in the cells. A feedback system maintains this fluid imbalance by the concentration of particles dissolved in the body's water. This is referred to as the "osmolality" of a solution and nutrients like glucose, salts, and minerals affect fluid balance. Think of osmolality of a fluid as a way for the water to move around, either getting pushed or pulled into or out of cells. For example, an energy drink is much more concentrated in sugar than a sports drink and some particles, like glucose, have more power to pull water around. Sodium and electrolytes contribute a small amount to the overall osmolality of the sports drink as well. Therefore, the greater the osmolaltiy of sugary drinks, the more likely an imbalance in water concentration can occur. Ideally, you want fluids during exercise to be closer to the body's own osmolality to expedite gastric emptying and delivery to tissues where it's needed. The proper balance of sugar and electrolytes facilitates proper fluid balance needed during training. Water, various sugars, and sodium and other electrolytes work in concert for optimal hydration. Although its reputation is tainted, sodium is an important nutrient during intense exercise, especially for athletes exercising in the heat or for long duration.

Maintaining blood volume is of prime importance to fluid balance. Various hormones along with organs such as the kidneys, adrenal glands, lungs, pituitary gland and hypothalamus play a role in fluid balance and regulation. The role of these various regulators is to tell the body to hold on to water and sodium or excrete water or sodium. The thirst reflex also helps regulate blood volume and is affected by the concentration of sodium in the body. If fluids shift, a chain of events occurs to include either a decrease in blood volume (dehydration) or an increase in blood volume (overhydration). Here are a few examples of athletes and fluid balance concerns:

Andy, Ironman athlete (low blood volume, dehydrated), heavy sweater

IN: 12 oz sports drink per hour, three-hour bike ride - inadequate fluid and sodium intake during exercise

OUT: fluid and sodium loss via sweat, minimal urine production

In this instance, low fluid volume and higher sodium concentrations signals the body to dilute the sodium level by retaining water via kidneys and borrowing water from other compartments. The thrist reflex kicks in, signaling the desire to drink. This effect can occur with as little as a two percent loss of body fluids. If water isn't replaced, stress on the heart, brain, and muscles increase and affect performance.

Nick, High School Football player (high blood volume, overhydrated), heavy sweater

IN: 48 ounces plain water bottle per hour, two hours practice (am & pm), Two– a -days

OUT: fluids and sodium loss via sweat, high urine production

Here, high fluid volume and lower sodium concentrations in the blood signal the body to concentrate sodium by increasing urination via the kidneys. Hands are swollen and stomach feels bloated. The thirst reflex shuts down and with it, the desire to drink. High intake of low or sodium-free drinks can shift the fluids out of the blood into spaces it does not belong.

Daily Fluid Balance

IN	OUT
Fluids (8 cups)	Urine (7 cups)
Foods (2 cups)	Skin/sweat (3 cups)
Metabolism (1.25 cups)	Lungs/Breathing (1.25 cups)
	Feces (.5 cups)
Total Intake: ~ 11 cups	Total Output: ~ 11 cups

Fluid Imbalance

It is not uncommon for athletes to show up to training dehydrated and usually do not drink adequate fluids during training as well. Hydration status needs to be addressed continuously, especially before (usually 24 hours) training begins. If neglected the athlete increases the risk of being chronically dehydrated and increasing the risk of injury and illness, fatigue, and poor performance.

Runners placed under heat stress were evaluated for drinking behavior and their perception of fluid needs versus actual consumption. They were given access to sports drinks *ad lib*. Results showed that they were found to have underestimated their sweat loss by 42% and only have replaced 30%. In a study of NCAA collegiate athletes, 138 males and 125 females, researchers assessed pre-practice hydration status, measuring urine specific gravity which measures the concentration of urine. Results showed only 34 percent appeared hydrated, with a mean urine specific gravity of 1.012 (see chart below). Another study on high school football players during preseason practices showed they replaced two-thirds of their sweat losses and were only mildly dehydrated. However, they did not adequately rehydrated between practices – a problem that ultimately affects performance. In another study, a group of NBA basketball players from five teams were evealuted for their hydration status. The researchers looked at the relationship between pregame urine specific gravity and the volume of fluid consumed. Athletes were given access to fluid *ad lib* during each of two games. Approximately half of the players were hydrated (USG < 1.020) but most did not meet sweat losses with *ad lib* fluid intake. The average amount of fluid consumed during the game was less than half of the volume required to match sweat losses. What impact does this have on performance? **Studies show that as little as a 2% fluid loss can impair performance. In fact, a 3% loss of body fluids can cause a 10% loss of strength and an 8% loss in speed.**

National Athletic Trainers Association – Dehydration Cutoffs

- Well Hydrated: Urine Specific Gravity (USG) < 1.010

- Minimally Dehydrated: USG 1.010-1.020

- Significantly Dehydrated: USG 1.020-1.030

- Seriously Dehydrated: USG > 1.030

Note: 1.021 and 1.030 may reflect 3% to 5% dehydration

Sweat & Electrolytes

Exercise produces heat that, unless released, can lead to significant increases in body temperature. Sweating is the body's primary means of releasing heat. Sweat evaporates from the skin and carries away the heat from working muscles. In fact, sweat evaporation is responsible for up to 80% of total heat loss. Only sweat that has evaporated has a cooling effect. If conditions are very humid or temperatures are mild, very little evaporation takes place. For example, sweating accounts for 20% of total heat lost at 50 degrees Fahrenheit but increases to 70% at 86 degrees Fahrenheit. As core body temperature increases so does the volume of sweat, which increases the risk of dehydration if fluids are not replaced. Dehydration thickens the blood due to decreased blood plasma volume and strains the cardiovascular system to maintain blood flow to exercising muscles. Athletes can decrease this risk by consuming adequate fluids and electrolytes. Coaches can help decrease the risk of dehydration by measuring the interaction of four environmental factors: air temperature, relative humidity, wind, and sun radiation. A device known as the wet-bulb globe temperature (WBGT) thermometer facilitates these measurements. Another indicator is the heat index, which combines air temperature and relative humidity.

- **Signs and Symptoms of dehydration**: confusion, weakness, increased heart rate, dizziness, headaches, nausea, chills, decreased sweating and higher rate of perceived rate of effort, Dark yellow urine

Sweat is 99 % water and 1% representing other substances including electrolytes such as sodium, chloride, calcium, magnesium, and potassium and smaller amounts of other minerals. Sweat rate (the volume sweat produced) and sweat composition will vary for each person and is influenced by a number of factors including exercise intensity, duration, environmental conditions and the type of clothing worn. Furthermore, individual characteristics such as body weight, genetics, heat acclimatization, gender and fitness level may impact how one sweats as well. Therefore, a one-size-fits-all hydration plan is inappropriate. Monitoring urine color and conducting sweat rates in different environments, different intensities and different sports will help dial in your hydration needs. Even though most coaches, athletes and trainers may not be able to measure urine specific gravity, they can monitor hydration by trending morning body weights and assessing urine color.

Electrolyte Sweat composition (average):

Sodium	**800-900 mg/L**
Potassium	150-200 mg/L
Calcium	30-40 mg/L
Magnesium	10-20 mg/L
Chloride	1000 mg/L

*Note: sodium concentration can vary (230-2300 mg/L)

Sodium Levels in fluids composition (average)

Type	Sodium	Carbohydrate (8 oz)
Regular*	440 mg/L	14 g
Endurance (high sodium)*	800 mg/L	14-17 g
Low sodium*	80 mg/L	14 g
Tomato Juice	2800 mg/L	10 g
Blood:		
Hyponatremia (115 meq/L)	2645 mg/L	X
Normal (135-145 meq/L)	3105-3335 mg/L	X
Sodium in Ocean Water	13,000 mg/L	X

*Sports drink

Electrolytes include sodium, potassium, calcium, magnesium, and chloride and are equally important as water itself. Not only do they affect fluid balance, they play a role conducting electrical impulses. Muscles and neurons rely on electrolytes for activity. Muscle contraction is dependent upon the presence of calcium, sodium, and potassium. The table below details each major electrolyte and its primary function for athletes. Out of all the electrolytes, sodium is the key electrolyte to monitor during training sessions because it is extensively lost during intense exercise.

Electrolyte	Function
Sodium	Critical for nerve transmission and muscle contraction, component of sodium bicarbonate – used as natural buffer for lactic acid

Electrolyte	Function
Potassium	Team up with sodium and chloride to regulate fluids, generate impulses in the nerves and muscles (i.e. heart). Helps carry glucose into muscle cells, helps storage of glycogen (i.e. muscle fuel)
Calcium	Muscle contraction, bone health, blood pressure, blood clotting, nerve transmission
Magnesium	Muscle contraction/relaxation, in > 300 enzymes, bone health, energy metabolism
Chloride	Team up with sodium to regulate fluids, helps form hydrochloric acid in the stomach to digest protein, communicator between cells

Sweat rate calculation:

Weigh with minimal clothing (before & after)
Record type of fluids, environmental conditions, training

1. Weight before exercise _____ -- Weight after exercise _____ = _____ lb
2. Weight difference in lbs (step 1) x 16 oz = _____ oz
3. Amount of fluids consumed during activity + _____ oz = Total fluids lost
4. Duration of activity = _____ hrs.
5. Sweat Rate = _____ / _____ = _____ oz per hr

Sample sweat rate: 175 lb – 172 lb = 3 lbs
3 lbs x 16 oz = 48 oz
20 oz fluids (sports drink) consumed, add to 48 oz
2 hrs (note: mild temperature, cloudy)
Sweat rate = 68 oz / 2 hrs = 34 oz/hr

Body weight lost as sweat	Physiological Effect
>2%	Impaired performance – endurance ↓ Mental performance
3%-5% 4%	Capacity for muscular strength/power may decline in heat Impair performance – endurance, cold weather
5%	Heat exhaustion - endurance
7%	Hallucinations
10%	Circulatory collapse and heat stroke

Fluid Imbalance:
Cardiac Stress, Heat Illnesses, and Muscle Cramps

When the blood volume decreases, the heart suffers. Heart rate increases, cardiac output – the amount of blood pumped per minute - drops and blood pressure decreases. Called "heat illnesses," the most common symptoms among athletes are heat cramps, heat syncope, and heat exhaustion.

Heat cramps: common in individuals who have lost a large amount of sweat, consumed a large amount of low sodium fluids, and who have excreted a small amount of urine.

Heat syncope (i.e. fainting) common during the first three to five days of heat exposure in non-acclimatized athletes exercising in a hot environment. The incidence of heat syncope is nearly zero after those three to five days in acclimatized athletes.

Heat exhaustion: most commonly diagnosed form of heat illness among athletes.

The benefits of heat acclimatization will start to disappear after only a few days or weeks of inactivity (about two to four weeks). The rate of loss depends on the number of heat exposures per week, the number and type of training sessions, and the degree to which core body temperature was raised. Interestingly, athletes with high VO2max values usually do not lose the adaptations of heat acclimatization as fast as individuals with a lower VO2max.

Muscle Cramps

No one knows for sure what causes muscle cramps: lack of stretching, nutrient deficiency, change in temperature, muscle fatigue, fitness level, dehydration, imbalance of electrolytes and fluids. So, if you have healthy kidneys and are not salt sensitive (i.e. high blood pressure) and all the exercise strategies have not worked – go for the salt (1/4-1/2 tsp per 24 oz sports drink) and look for sporst drinks that add some magnesium, calcium and potassium.

Electrolyte Imbalance: Hyponatremia

Hyponatremia is a metabolic condition in which there is not enough sodium (salt) in the body fluids outside the cells. Women typically have lower sweat rates and electrolyte losses than men due to smaller body size. However, women are at greater risk of exercise-associated hyponatremia, especially less fit individuals. A major cause of hyponatremia is drinking fluids low in sodium, such as water, beyond the amount needed to replace sweat loss. In general, risk for hyponatremia increases when exercising less than four hours and consuming excessive amounts of low-sodium fluids. Training greater than four hours, the sodium losses alone can place the athlete at risk.

Signs and Symptoms (based on blood levels)

If sodium levels in the blood drop below 130 mmol/L to 125 mmol/L , symptoms include headache, vomiting, swollen hands and feet, fatigue, confusion, and disorientation and wheezy breathing. At less than 120 mmol/L, cerebral edema, seizures, coma, and even death can occur.

Rhabdomyolsis

A syndrome caused by severe exertion during training that results in the release of muscle tissue breakdown markers into the blood such as creatine kinase. Clinically, rhabdomyolsis is defined as having creatine kinase levels greater than 10 times normal. Cases have been found in training academies, such as police or the military. Even though it is not common, coaches and trainers need to be aware of the possible health effects of excessive muscle damage and dehydration. Myoglobin, a component of muscle tissue, is released into the blood and could affect kidney function as well. Dead muscle tissue may cause a large amount of fluid to move from the blood into the muscle, reducing fluid volume and leading to shock. Reduced blood flow can have a tremendous impact on the kidneys as a state of dehydration increases the risk of renal failure.

Fluid Plans:

Fluids before training

Timing	Volume	Fluid Type
>3-4 hr	2 cups or 5-7 ml/kg* (select based on the ability to produce urine)	Fluids (carbs, moderate pro, low fat): juice, sports drinks Sodium (450-1150 mg/L)
2 hr	2 cups or 3-5** ml/kg	Sports drink 4-8% Sodium (~500 ml)
10-15 min	1 cup	Water/sports drink

ACSM guidelines (2007): if unable to produce urine*, drink again** to allow urine output to return to normal

Fluid Replacement needs during activity:

Total Sweat Rate _____ oz / hr (from calculation)

Determine the number of times you will drink per hour to achieve at least 80% of your sweat rate.

Example: every 10 min, drink 3-4 sips/swallows (ie ~1 swallow = 1 oz) or five to six swallows every 15 minutes.

Training	Timing	Total Volume/hr	Fluid Type
< 1 hr	Every 10-20 min.	13-28+ oz/hr (400-800 ml)*	Water Sports Drink *(optional, unless you have not consumed snack/meal past 3-4 hrs)*

Training	Timing	Total Volume/hr	Fluid Type
> 1 hr	Every 10-20 min.	13-28+ oz/hr (400-800 ml)*	Sports drink (11-19 gm carbohydrate/8 oz) or 4-8% Sodium (~500-1000 mg/L)* Potassium (80-200 mg/L)
Marathon Runners**	2-6 hrs	13-26 oz (400 -800 ml/hr)*	Sports drink (11-19 gm carbohydrate/8 oz) or 4-8% Sodium (~500-1000 mg/L)* Potassium (80-200 mg/L)

*Dependent on sweat rate. **ACSM (2007)

Gastric (stomach) emptying

Two main factors affect the speed at which dietary fluids get into the body: speed of gastric emptying and rate of absorption from the small intestine. Other factors include carbohydrate amount in the fluid, dehydration, increased core temperature. High intensity exercise (80-85% maximum heart rate) will slow or even stop gastric emptying. For athletes, sports drinks supply an appropriate sugar concentration (4 to 8% or 4 to 8 g per 100 ml) so that fluids can pass quickly through the gut, empty into the small intestine and finally into the blood for transport to working muscles. Sodium in a sports drink will reduce urine output, enable the fluid to empty quickly from the stomach, promote absorption from the intestine and encourage fluid retention. Exercise intensity up to 75 % maximum heart rate has little effect on gastric emptying. By the way, cold drinks are not absorbed into your body more quickly than warm ones.

Just as we can train our muscles and cardiovascular system, we can train the gut too! Practice with different products (liquids/solids/chews/gels), concentrations of sugars, sodium and fluid during training and allow enough time for the body and gut to adapt. Never try anything new on competition day.

Optional: Acute Sodium loading

It has been shown athletes can hyper-hydrate before an event by consuming extra sodium pre-exercise. A study with 13 female cyclists riding in 90 degree heat, 50% RH, consuming a low sodium drink (230 milligrams/L) or high sodium drink (3772 milligrams/L) over 105 minutes before exercise confirms this. The results showed a pre-exercise ingestion of high sodium drink increased blood volume, reduced thermoregulatory strain, and increased exercise capacity. They were able to ride 20% longer. Sodium acts like a sponge to attract and hold on to water in the blood.

Recovery/Post-Training

Timing	Volume	Fluid Type
Start as soon as practical,	23 oz/1 lb body wt lost	Sports drink (11-19 gm carbohydrate/8 oz) or 4-8% Sodium (~500-1000 mg/L) Potassium (80-200 mg/L) Protein 20-30 g + solid foods as desired
Eat/drink within 2 hr, repeat again in 6 hr recovery window	Check urine color & weight	

According to ACSM's position on exercise and fluid replacement, consuming sodium in the recovery period will help retain ingested fluids along with stimulating thirst. Another nutrient shown to enhance fluid retention is protein because it too, acts like a magnet to hold on to water. When a "binding" agent such as sodium or protein is lacking in a beverage and the athlete chooses to drink just plain water (such as wanting to lower calories for weight loss), they have missed out. The body will use some of the fluids to put back into the cells, but most will be lost in the urine.

Heat Acclimatization

Competing in a hot environment presents special considerations because of the increased risk of dehydration and fatigue as well as your health concerns. Regulation of body temperature during exercise in the heat is critical and proper hydration plays a major role in that process. Heat is hard to beat and if the body is not prepared - either through training adaptations and/or lacking fluids – the risk for heat illnesses increases. Heat acclimatization is a planned training strategy that builds your tolerance to heat over a period of time, typically 10 to 14 days. During this time the athlete undergoes repeated bouts of exercise in a hot environment. The body adapts to the heat stress by making changes in sweat rate, sweat composition (i.e. conserves sodium) and the cardiovascular system (i.e. lower heart rate). These changes result in better control of core body temperature. Benefits can be felt in the first one to five days. Physiologically, a three to twenty-seven percent increase in plasma volume is seen due to higher retention of plasma proteins and sodium in the blood. Heart rate decreases 15 percent to 25 percent. Additional benefits include increase in blood flow to the skin, increased blood volume, and possibly a sparing of glycogen.

Changes	Number of Days
↓ Perceived exertion decrease	3-5 days
↓ Heart Rate Decrease	3-6 days
↑ Blood/Plasma volume	
↓ Kidney sodium and Chloride concentration	3-8 days
↓ Core temp	5-8 days
↓ Sweat sodium and Chloride concentration	5-10 days
↑ Sweat Na+ and Sweat rate	8-14 days

Cold Environment

Cold environments can pose a threat to the hydration levels of endurance athletes as well since cold air can increase water loss and augment dehydration. Athletes drink too little fluids in cold weather because the thirst reflex is diminished. Urine output is increased with cold environmental exposure. Cold air also contains less water vapor and leads to increased water loss. More water is also needed by the body to warm and moisturize cold, dry air breathed into the lungs.

Altitude

Water loss is increased significantly at higher altitude due to increased water loss from respiration and an increased urinary water loss due to a change in a hormone regulation. The water loss from the lungs alone is three to four times higher than an individual at lower altitude. Water loss ranges from eight cups per day for men and three and one-half cups per day for women. Urinary water loss can be as high as two cups. This equates to about 2.4 liters/day for men and 1.35 liters/day for women.

Air Travel

Air travel effects hydration status much like altitude. Airplane cabins are pressurized to 6000 to 9000 feet and the relative humidity can be as low as one percent. Water loss from being in this low relative humidity adds up to water loss as high as three to four cups above normal. Drink you fluids when flying!

Urine Color Chart

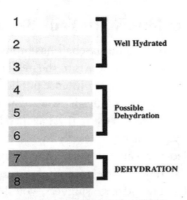

Collect sample in clear plastic container.
Hold up to bright light for comparison.

The urine color chart is reproduced with permission from Lawrence Armstrong and Human Kinetics and was originally published in Lawrence Armstrong's book titled *Performing in Extreme Environments*. The book may be purchased from Human Kinetics by calling (800) 747-4457 or online at www.humankinetics.com

CHAPTER 8

Steroids/Precursor Hormones/
Banned Substances: Playing Russian
Roulette With Your Body

Playing Russian Roulette With Your Body

The 'Steroid Era' in Major League Baseball has brought the use of illegal performance-enhancing drugs in sports to the media forefront. With this dawning of an ominous era there has been intense public debate as to whether or not using performance enhancing drugs is ethically wrong and/or whether or not there are negative side effects to using these agents. Notably, our current vice president Joe Biden (who has been heavily involved in architecting anti-steroid legislation) has led the vehement scolding of baseball players that purportedly used steroids. If you were to compare the statistics of 1970's sluggers versus late 1990's 'Steroid Era' sluggers, you'll likely find that the latter players (on average) hit double the amount of home-runs per 500 at-bats; this being a phenomenon which is in line with vice president Biden's notion that steroid users are cheating. Numerous research laboratories, however, have performed clinical research in elder and/or critically ill persons which illuminates the positives benefits of administering steroids as medicinal means of hormone therapy; notably, increased muscle mass, increased strength, increased energy levels, and increased quality of life. What further obscures the debate about steroid use is the recent push from pharmaceutical companies who are aggressively marketing testosterone therapy to older males. According to advertisements, steroid therapy will likely improve fatigue, reduced libido, depression, muscle mass, fat mass, and bone mass in the estimated 13 million

Americans that have lower than normal testosterone levels; note that the same can also be said for a post-menopausal woman popping estrogen pills (the female steroid) on a daily basis. And then there is even newer research pushing steroid therapy on women as a means of increasing energy and sexual drive - is there any wonder as to why there exists massive confusion about the issue about steroid use in society?!?

A Grey Area

The truth about steroids is that there are two sides to the story which are well blended by an obscure grey area. On one end of the spectrum is the undeniable fact that steroids confer positive benefits in users. In fact, the reason why several professional athletes have resorted to using illegal performance enhancing drugs is the very reason that their name implies... these compounds give athletes an unfair advantage compared to non-users. On the other end of the spectrum is fact that they're illegal, banned in sports, and will likely lead to one or multiple negative side effects. The grey area is extended to the vast sports nutrition market whereby many companies claim that their products are the legal and just-as-effective alternatives to illegal performance enhancing drugs. While there are indeed safe and effective over-the-counter nutritional supplements that increase athletic performance as well as companies that ensure rigorous quality control standards, there is also the other proverbial side of the coin in which potential problems can arise when consuming unsubstantiated over-the-counter supplements. Specifically, some products: a) may be contaminated with a substance that could cause a negative health effect, b) may contain an ingredient that causes the athlete to fail a drug screening, or c) may contain a compound that is very similar to illegal drugs and could potentially cause negative health effects with long-term use. Therefore, every coach, athlete, and parent should be aware about which popular legal and illegal performance-enhancing agents exist, how these agents purportedly work, and how abusing these compounds will likely lead to one or multiple deleterious health consequences. More importantly, the end of this chapter will give tips as to how patrons can protect themselves from consuming over-the-counter ingredients that may negatively affect his/her health.

ANABOLIC STEROIDS

History. Relative to the field of sports nutrition, which was thought to exist with the ancient Olympians, steroids have had a brief history. In 1935 scientists isolated testosterone from testicular extracts and, soon thereafter in 1939, German chemists Adolf Butenandt and Leopold Ruzicka developed laboratory methods for synthesizing testosterone; this being a feat that earned both scholars the Nobel Prize in Chemistry. The muscle strengthening and rejuvenating properties of testosterone led the Soviets to aggressively push steroid drug schedules on their weightlifting athletes in the 1940s. It wasn't until the mid 1950s that the Americans caught on. Touted as the "Doctor who brought steroids to America", Dr. John Ziegler attended the 1954 World Weightlifting Championships in Austria as the team's physician. He noted the athletic superiority of the Soviets and purportedly told the Los Angeles Times in a subsequent interview that *"some of the competitors, even young ones in their 20s, needed to be catheterized in order to urinate"*. His observation was likely that of prostate growth in the Soviet athletes which is indicative of steroid abuse. Regardless, Ziegler returned to the states and spearheaded the late 1950's production of an oral testosterone analog named methandrostenolone (i.e., Dianabol or D-bol). Therein the official 'steroid era' in sports fervently ensued between the Americans and Soviets and it quickly blossomed to other countries. By 1976, 2 out of 3 Olympic athletes had anonymously admitted to steroid use, despite the fact that only 8% of the tested athletes tested positive for them, and anecdotal reports suggested that up to 90% of NFL players were steroid users in the 1970's!

Steroids became banned from international competition by the International Olympic Committee in 1976 and, because it was apparent that several athletes self-administered steroids during training and not during competition, the advent of routine drug screening occurred nearly a decade later. It wasn't until the late1980's that the United States law-makers decided to intervene and combat the fervent use of steroids in American sports with legislation. Congressional hearings between 1988 and 1990 led to the implementation of the Anabolic Steroids Control Act of 1990 which declared:

- Anabolic steroids were grouped in the same legal category as other drugs (i.e., a Schedule III drug) such as tranquilizers, amphetamines and morphine to mention a few.

- Possessing steroids became a federal offense and was punishable with a minimum fine of $1,000 as well as up to a one year prison sentence. Individuals caught possessing steroids that had been previously convicted of possessing drugs (i.e., repeat offenders) would receive a prison sentence of 15 days to 2 years as well as minimum $2,500 fine. Triple possession offenders would receive 90 days to 3 years in prison as well as a minimum $5,000 fine.

- Persons who sold, or possessed with the intent to sell (i.e., were caught with an amount that is deemed more than for personal use) could receive up to 5 years of imprisonment and/or a $250,000 fine. Repeat offenders could be sentenced to 10 years of prison and/or larger fines.

While this legislation made it more difficult to obtain steroids, dangerous underground practices became common in order to fulfill the demand for these drugs. Specifically, many steroids were and still are: a) manufactured by pharmaceutical companies outside the U.S. and smuggled through the mail, b) manufactured legally in the U.S. and diverted to the black market, or c) illegally home-cooked. It is also common that anabolic steroids supplied on the black market can be diluted, contaminated and unsterile, and/or counterfeited. Nevertheless, steroid abuse is still purportedly prevalent from the high school to collegiate to professional athlete

Steroids Mechanisms of Muscle Action

Chemists design anabolic steroids with the intent of mimicking the physiological effects of testosterone. Briefly, testosterone is a cholesterol-based sex steroid produced in the testes of males and (to a marginal degree) in the ovaries of females and it is the hormone responsible for the gender differences in muscle mass and strength. There are several ways in which testosterone and steroids are thought to increase muscle mass and strength (Figure 8). Clinical trials have demonstrated that administering very high doses of testosterone to younger and older men markedly increases muscle mass and strength as well as circulating 'free' testosterone, the number of resident stem cells in skeletal muscle, and the average size of mature muscle cells. This has led to the belief that steroid-induced increases in muscle size and strength are due to steroids causing the addition of muscle stem cells to previous mature muscle cells which increases gross muscle size. The end result is larger muscles with stronger contractile capabilities and that strength gains are amplified through increases in size of nerves that communicate with muscle cells and 'tell' them to contract. Others hypothesize that steroids are able to signal the muscle to 'build' more muscle proteins which amplifies strength and muscle mass. Unfortunately, the long-term effects on muscle repair mechanisms with steroid use are unknown and potentially hazardous given that steroids signal the usage of valuable muscle stem cells that are important for muscle repair during aging.

Thus, it is apparent that steroid users have an unfair athletic advantage to non-users due to the drastic increases in strength and muscle mass these individuals incur during self-administration even though little is known at the neuromuscular level what can or will happen with prolonged use.

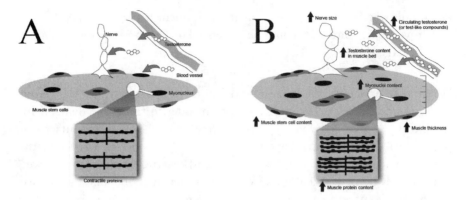

Steroids are typically administered orally or are injected intramuscularly. Oral agents are typically taken on a daily or semi-daily basis due to the fact that the active compound is broken down expeditiously by the liver during digestion. Injectable steroids are typically administered once or twice weekly and hang around much longer in circulation because: a) it takes longer for the compound to dissipate from the injection spot and b) several injectable compounds are tagged with long-acting esters (i.e., enanthate or decanoate as examples). There are numerous steroid variants (or analogs) that share chemical properties with testosterone. Steroid analogs are created with the intent of: a) optimizing the muscle-building effects while trying to minimize the negative side effects, b) extending the duration the compound circulates in the blood, or c) making a compound that is resilient to drug screenings (as with 'the Clear' or THG prior to the B.A.L.C.O. Scandal (discussed later). Nonetheless, the Anabolic Steroid Control Acts of 1988 and 2004 have deemed the use of all steroid analogs illegal and, to date, there has not been the creation of an analog that yields solely positive gains without negative side effects. In this regard, users often resort to taking other drugs in an attempt to remedy negative side effects incurred. For example, users that are sensitive to estrogenic effects of steroids (i.e., water retention and/or the development of gynecomastia) will commonly self-administer estrogen receptor blockers (i.e., Tamoxifen) or aromatase inhibitors (i.e, Anastrozole, Letrozole) in an attempt to combat these undesired effects. Users that are sensitive to the androgenic effects of steroids such as acne and/or hair loss may try to slow the progression of these effects with the concomitant administration of a 5α-reductase inhibitor (i.e., Finasteride). Users will also commonly administer post-cycle agents (i.e., hCG or Clomiphene) in an attempt to re-coup their natural testosterone production or other compounds in an attempt to lose excess body fat that they may have incurred during their cycle (i.e., clenbuterol); this practice is termed **post-cycle therapy**). Finally, it should be mentioned that steroid users will commonly combine testosterone analogs during a cycle (termed **stacking**) in an attempt to obtain synergistic effects from various drug combinations. For instance, it is anecdotally purported that stacking the oral analog D-bol with injectable drugs (i.e., testosterone and/ or nandrolone esters) optimizes strength gains during the early part of the cycle. In summary, many users resort to becoming a walking pharmaceutical depot in order to try to maximize the positive benefits of steroid use while trying to prevent the body from negatively reacting to these drugs. Table 1 lists common testosterone analogs as well as other ancillary drugs used during or after a steroid cycle.

Table 1. Common steroids or other compounds used in conjunction with a steroid cycle

Analogs (trade name)	Properties	Structure
Testosterone esters	Injectable oil commonly stored in 10 ml vials or small ampoules Tagged with esters at –OH position to affect ½ life in circulation (i.e., acetate, cypionate, enanthate)	
Nandrolone decanoate (Deca) or Nandrolone phenylpropionate	Injectable oil commonly stored in 10 ml vials or small ampoules Tagged with a 10-carbon ester at –OH position to increase ½ life in circulation	
Methyltestosterone	Oral (tab form) User can experience exaggerated 'androgenic' side effects (i.e., headaches, increased blood pressure, irritability) and rapid weight gain	
Trenbolone acetate (Finaplix) or enanthate	Injectable oil commonly stored in 10 ml vials or small ampoules Tagged with acetate or enanthate ester at –OH position to increase ½ life in circulation Gynecomastia can ensue due to its progesterone receptor binding affinity	
Oxandrolone (Anavar)	Oral (tab form) Anecdotally side effects are more mild than other agents making it popular with female athletes	

Methandrostenolone (Dianabol or D-bol)	Oral(tab form) User can experience exaggerated 'androgenic' side effects (i.e., headaches, increased blood pressure, irritability) and rapid weight gain within days of use	
Boldenone undecylenate (Equipoise)	Injectable oil commonly stored in 10 ml vials or small ampoules Tagged with a 10-carbon ester at –OH position to increase ½ life in circulation Anecdotally side effects are more mild than other agents making it popular with female athletes	
Stanozolol (Winstrol)	Oral (tab form) or water-based injectable Anecdotally side effects are more mild than other agents making it popular with female athletes	
Oxymethelone (Anadrol 50)	Oral (tab form) User can experience exaggerated 'androgenic' side effects (i.e., headaches, increased blood pressure, irritability) and rapid weight gain within days of use	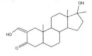

Other commons agents used during or after steroid cycle

Tamoxifen (Nolvadex)	Oral (tab form) Estrogen receptor blocker taken in an attempt to offset 'estrogenic' effects (gynecomastia and water retention)
Anastrozole (Arimidex) or Letrozole (Femara)	Oral (tab form) Aromatase inhibitors (i.e., inhibit steroid conversion to estrogens) taken during a cycle in an attempt to offset 'estrogenic' effects (gynecomastia and water retention)
Human chorionic gonadotropin (hCG) or Clomiphene (Clomid)	hCG is water-based injectable commonly stored in ampoules, Clomid is oral (tab form) Used to at the end of and after a cycle to try to recoup natural testosterone production
Finasteride (Propecia or Proscar)	Oral (tab form) 5α-reductase inhibitors (i.e., inhibit steroid conversion to DHT-like compounds) taken during a cycle in an attempt to offset 'androgenic' effects (i.e., acne, hair loss, and irritability)

Physiological dangers of steroid abuse

There are grave physiological consequences that can ensue with steroid abuse. While there are swift increases in strength and muscle mass, scientists have revealed that other dangerous side effects (some irreversible) commonly occur with prolonged use (summarized in Table 2).

Table 2. Researched side effects of prolonged steroid abuse

Side effects of prolonged steroid abuse	Reversible
Endocrine disorders	
Gynecomastia in males (i.e., development of male breast tissue)	**No, requires surgery**
Testicular atrophy and decreased sperm production	Yes
Cardiovascular	
Ventricular hypertrophy (i.e., pathologic heart growth)	Not known
Increase in blood pressure	Yes
Blood thickening	Yes
Decrease in good cholesterol and an increase in bad cholesterol	Yes
Brain function	
Chemical dependence and addiction	Yes if discontinued
Aggression (increases with duration of use)	Yes
Post-cycle depression in some users	Yes
Dermatological	
Acne (can vary in degree of severity)	Permanent scarring can occur
Accelerates male pattern balding (only present in those predisposed to balding)	**No**
Bodily hair growth in males and females	Yes
Musculoskeletal	
Increased incidence of muscle and ligament injuries	Not known, injuries post-cycle have been reported
Premature growth plate fusion in adolescents (i.e., stunted growth)	**No**
Other reported side effects	
Fatty liver disease or liver damage (evidenced as jaundice)	Not known
Prostate growth and accelerated prostate cancer in those predisposed to the disease	Growth: Yes/ **Cancer: No**
Enlarged clitoris in females	**No**
Deepening of voice in females	**No**
Kidney failure (rare occurrence)	**No**
Impotence	Yes
Localized infection with injections (lack of sterility due to home-cooking or poor injection practices)	In rare cases, severe infection or abscesses can ensue

While the long-term effects of steroid abuse seem less daunting to users, there are immediate problems that users can encounter which are often debilitating. A well-known acute effect of steroid use includes an accelerated risk for soft-tissue injuries such as tendon and ligament tears due to the fact that: a) muscle growth during steroid cycles occurs at a disproportional rate to tendon and ligament growth and, b) an exaggerated amount of circulating steroids may mechanistically compromise connective tissue strength. Likewise, there are serious dermatological complications that can arise from steroid use as well. Finally, there is the risk for users that self-administer injectables to develop gruesome bacterial infections at injection sites due to poor sterilization techniques; this being anecdotally more common with counterfeited black market products or home-cooked products that aren't aseptically prepared. Internet steroid chat rooms are littered with stories similar to the aforementioned case.

Recent media attention

Illegal steroid use in sports has been under intense media and public scrutiny and what became known as the 'B.A.L.C.O. Scandal' undoubtedly ignited it. From 2002-2003, the IRS and U.S. Doping Agency had Victor Conte and his company the Bay Area Laboratory Cooperative in their crosshairs for money laundering and steroid trafficking. On September 3, 2003 an invasion on the premises confirmed the latter suspicions and subsequent raids yielded the drug schedules of several high profile U.S. athletes which suggested that they had frequented Conte's facilities for the purpose of illegally obtaining steroids. Notably, allegations arose that Major League Baseball's Barry Bonds had been given a previously undetectable steroid named tetrahydrogestrinone (referred to as THG or 'the Clear') the year during and prior to him setting the MLB record for home runs in a single season. Olympic champion and female sprinter Marion Jones was another beloved athlete revealed as one of many Conte's clients. Following her 2007 admission to knowingly taking steroids, Jones was stripped of her Olympic medals and consequently served 6 months of prison for perjury. Bonds has admitted that he unknowingly took 'the Clear' supplied by B.A.L.C.O.'s trainer Greg Anderson.

Beyond the high profile cases of Barry Bonds and Marion Jones, the domino effect that ensued following the B.A.L.C.O. scandal was widespread. In response to the negative press that Bonds received as well as speculation that other players were using steroids, Commissioner Bud Selig recruited U.S. Senator George Mitchell to investigate the illegal use of steroids and human growth hormone (or hGH) in Major League Baseball. In 2007 Senator Mitchell released a 400+ page document (dubbed the Mitchell Report) which cited evidence suggesting that 89 former and current players illegally used steroids as means of bolstering sports performance. Pitcher Roger Clemens was one of the incriminated players tarnished during these proceedings and, like Bonds, he denies knowingly using steroids. In response to these proceedings, Major League Baseball has revised its substance abuse policy to carry harsher penalties for players that fail steroid drug tests. The NFL came under post B.A.L.C.O. fire as well. In 2005, Jason Scukanec (formerly of Brigham Young's college football team) came forward and discussed the prevalence of steroid use in college football estimating that the 'more temperate' BYU program had up to 20 users on the team. Scukanec went on to say in a Portland, Oregon newspaper interview:

"My best friend was a steroid monster... He was naturally 245 or 250 pounds, but he got up to 312 with a 36-inch waist. He had stretch marks on his chest and shoulder and eventually blew out both of his knees... Another guy we played with, who is still in the NFL, would come back at the end of a season weighing 270. Three weeks into the offseason, he was 295 and buffed. It wasn't a big mystery what he was doing. Three guys I played with in the NFL, I saw them use. The coaches knew the guys on the juice. To pretend it doesn't go on would be a farce. It's the big 'no-no' nobody wants to talk about. And you don't want to know what's going on at the junior college level, where no testing is being done."

To date, former NFL All Pro and B.A.L.C.O. client Dana Stubblefield is the one of only a handful of football players to be incriminated in the B.A.L.C.O. Scandal and received 2 years of probation. In 2008 the San Diego Tribune subsequently performed what they touted as an NFL equivalent to the Mitchell Report and unveiled nearly 100 professional football players dating back to the 1960's that had used steroids and/or other banned performance enhancers.

Public policy also changed in response to the 'B.A.L.C.O. Scandal'. Current vice president Joseph Biden spearheaded legislation that led to the Anabolic Steroid Control Act of 2004 which amended previous steroid legislation by banning over-the-counter sales of nearly 40 prohormones (except for dehydroepiandrosterone or DHEA) and scheduled them as controlled substances. Furthermore, this act annually pledged (between 2005-2010) $15 million in order to fund entities to educate children in elementary and secondary schools about the harmful effects of anabolic steroids. Additionally, $1 million was devoted annually to the National Survey on Drug Use and Health so that it includes questions concerning the use of anabolic steroids. Nevertheless, The use of steroids and banned substances from high school on up is becoming a major problem for all. The Center for Disease Control and Prevention's (CDC) Youth Risk Behavior Surveillance reported that the percentage of students who reported steroid use during 2005 was at approximately 4.0%. Other university surveys report up to approximately 3% of high school seniors have tried steroids at least once in their lifetime for the purposes of enhancing their performance in sports and to be more competitive in efforts to get an athletic scholarship. Unfortunately, the young athlete faces a host of potential problems with steroid use including increased aggression and irritability known as "roid rage", testicular atrophy (shrunken testicles), impotence, decreased sex drive, decreased mental and physical activity, lowering of good HDL (high density lipoprotein) cholesterol and an increase in bad LDL (low density lipoprotein) cholesterol, alterations in connective tissue structure which can weaken tendons, collagen fibers and reduce their strength and certain form of hepatitis (with a few cases of liver cancer reported.

Finally, large-scale steroid operations have been heavily persecuted since the breaking of the B.A.L.C.O. story in 2003. In 2007, the U.S. Drug Enforcement Agency was part of an international effort that ceased operations in nearly 60 steroid laboratories spanning 10 countries in an 18-month investigation named "Operation Raw Deal". Similarly, "Operation Gear Grinder" in 2005 aided in the downfall of major Mexican steroid manufacturers that used web-based means to distribute products to U.S. customers. All in all, the increased public and legislative awareness of illegal steroid use following the 'B.A.L.C.O. Scandal' has seemingly improved the prognosis of steroid use in general, although another wave of post-B.A.L.C.O. survey-based sports doping research will unveil the long-term success of these efforts.

Prohormones and Dangerous or Unsubstantiated over-the-counter Supplements

There largely exists a misconception that the supplement industry is not regulated in the United States. Renowned sport supplement Dr. Richard Kreider outlines the regulations as follows:

- Prior to 2006, manufacturers and distributors of dietary supplements were not required to record, investigate or communicate with the Food and Drug Administration (FDA) reports they received concerning injuries that were potentially related to the use of their products.

- In 2006, companies became required by the Dietary and Supplement and Nonprescription Drug Consumer Act to record all adverse event complaints about their products and make them available to the FDA within 15 days of the complaint. "Serious" adverse events include those which results in death, a life-threatening experience, inpatient hospitalization, a persistent or significant disability or incapacity, or a congenital anomaly or birth defect; or requires, based on a reasonable medical judgment, a medical or one which requires surgical intervention to prevent an outcome described above.

- Unfortunately, these reports can be false or unsubstantiated and can be blown out of proportion by the media; this has occurred in the past with creatine supplements which have been repeatedly deemed safe.

- The FDA has the authority to remove supplements from the marketplace if scientific evidence demonstrates that the supplement is unsafe; this was done with the publically controversial stimulant ephedra in 2004.

- The Federal Trade Commission (FTC) ensures that manufacturers are truthful and not misleading regarding claims they make about dietary supplements. The FTC also has the power to act against companies who make false and/or misleading marketing claims about a specific product. This includes acting against companies if the ingredients found in the supplement do not match label claims or in the event undeclared, drug ingredients are present (e.g., analogs of weight loss drugs or steroids as examples).

- These aforementioned measures provide a means for governmental oversight of the dietary supplement industry.

In spite of the aforementioned government regulations and the existence of ethical supplement companies there are over-the-counter supplements that: a) are not researched for safety and efficacy, and b) contain ingredients that may be potentially harmful with prolonged use. Furthermore, there have been cases where athletes fail drug screenings because he/she consumed a supplement containing a banned substance. Finally, there are also companies that, in spite of the Anabolic Control Steroid Act of 2004 which outlawed the sales of numerous prohormones, market newer generation prohormones that structurally resemble steroids and can carry similar ill side effects.

Prohormones. Prohormones are a class of compounds that bear an almost identical chemical resemblance to testosterone or other anabolic steroids, albeit many of these compounds have to be chemically converted by the body into more active compounds to experience steroid-like muscle-building effects (Figure 9); of note, negative side effects which will be discussed below are very common with prohormones.

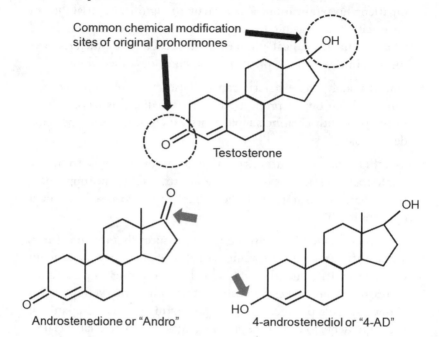

Figure 9. Examples of two popularly marketed prohormones (Andro and 4-AD) prior to their being scheduled as illegal drugs in 2004. This diagram illustrates the slight chemical alterations that prohormone manufacturers make in order to find legal loopholes for their distribution (red arrows). There is putative evidence that prohormones need to be converted by the body into the more powerful metabolite (for instance, 4-AD needs to be converted back into testosterone by enzymes in the testes in order to be effective). While the Anabolic Steroid Control Act of 2004 banned nearly 40 of these compounds, this practice still exists today.

Despite the fact that steroids were outlawed in 1988, prohormones made their way into the marketplace in 1996 when chemist and entrepreneur Patrick Arnold introduced androstenedione to the world; Arnold would later serve 3 months in prison for his role in designing THG for B.A.L.C.O.'s Victor Conte. Soon thereafter, the market became flooded with second generation legal steroid derivatives (i.e., 4-androstenediol, 1-androstenediol 1,4-androstadiendione as examples) that possessed a purportedly higher endogenous conversion rate into more active metabolites. However, what would become the fallout legislation following B.A.L.C.O. (i.e., the Anabolic

Control Steroid Act of 2004) illegalized the sales and manufacturing of nearly 40 of these compounds. While this legislation undoubtedly crippled numerous prohormone manufacturers, some companies began creatively crafting third generation prohormones that possessed legal chemical structural loopholes. Likewise, some companies began what would become the mass marketing of legal aromatase inhibitors. Briefly, these compounds purportedly shunt the endogenous production of estrogen in both sexes through the inhibition of the enzyme cytochrome p450 aromatase. In theory this would bolster testosterone levels given the fact that testosterone is a substrate of this enzyme (this is also why self-administering massive steroid or prohormone dosages can lead to estrogen build-up and unwanted estrogenic side effects). Research studies with over-the-counter aromatase inhibitors did reveal that large daily dosages (up to 600 mg per day) increased testosterone levels over weeks of supplementation in recreational bodybuilders, although there were also significant increases in circulating estrogen and DHT (a testosterone derivative associated with negative androgenic effects discussed above) with the use of a product called 6-OXO. Furthermore, these hormonal alterations did not translate into increases in muscle mass thus negating the effectiveness of these compounds.

To date, the sprouting of numerous over-the-counter prohormones has resurfaced, although the DEA is trying to keep up in scheduling them as drugs. Notably, in 2010 the DEA scheduled boldione, desoxymethyltestosterone (Madol), and 19-nor-4,9(10)-androstadienedione as illegal anabolic steroids in response to their widespread internet sales and prevalence in over-the-counter supplements prior to the ban. Unfortunately, however, there are supplement companies to date that continue to push the internet sales of next generation prohormones that have not been evaluated for safety and efficacy (examples of such products are shown in Figure 10).

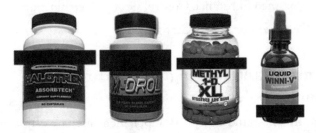

Figure 10. Supplement labels of some of the few currently marketed prohormones products on the internet.

As with steroid use, there have been numerous adverse events associated with using over-the-counter prohormones; notably, gynecomastia, accelerated male-patterned balding, increased blood pressure, negative alterations in blood lipids, and decrements in the body's own testosterone production. Unlike the use of illegal anabolic steroids, however, there is no scientific literature proving that legal prohormones are effective at increasing muscle mass and strength. A 2010 case study revealed that a 31-year-old man taking an over-the-counter prohormone supplement had become extremely irritable and developed a severe case of acute hepatitis; effects that disappeared after the supplement was discontinued. A similar case study in 2007 revealed that two young men developed what was termed as 'cholestatic liver panels' which required medical attention and was ultimately rectified following the discontinuation of these products. Finally, a review of the medical literature as of 2009 documented 6 cases of hepatotoxicity and one case of kidney failure associated with the use of prohormone-containing supplements. Of particular importance to athletes, supplements that possess prohormones in them can also lead to positive drug screenings. For the most part, the typical mainstream sports drinks, bars and powders produced by major food and dietary supplement companies are safe to use. Unfortunately, some of the unscrupulous small supplement manufacturers who specifically target the bodybuilding community have been suspect and many of the prohormones being sold have been documented to cause a positive doping result from the typical screening tests performed. In addition, the evidence suggests that the side effects from over-the-counter supplements containing prohormones can pose serious health threats to users.

Therefore, to ensure that consumers are well-protected and can enjoy products that are free of banned substances including steroids, hormones, prohormones, stimulants, etc., you will need to look on the label and marketing materials for the following seal of approvals:

- BSCG (Banned Substance Control Group) Certification
- NSF (Certified For Sport) Certification

Other unsubstantiated ingredients present in nutritional supplements

Beyond the muscle-building sports supplement arena exists a much more lucrative market of stimulant weight loss products that are sold to millions of customers on an annual basis. According to a recent estimation, weight loss stimulant products reap in an annual $37 billion world-wide. These stimulants have moved into the sports community under the guise of "thermogenic" agents. This market growth, however, is accompanied by the existence of unscrupulous companies that place unsubstantiated ingredients into their products. Briefly, the common goal of thermogenic supplements is to cause users to experience a decrease in body fat stores through an increase in fat breakdown and/or whole-body metabolism as well as the stimulant "buzz" targeted primarily to the young athletes.

Prior to its controversial ban by the FDA in 2004 ephedra-based supplements had been shown to facilitate short-term weight loss in clinical trials. The putative cardiovascular side effects of ephedra, some which were scientifically-proven and presented in the New England Journal of Medicine and some which were largely media-driven, was brought to the government's attention thus cinching the banning of ephedra-containing products. As with the prohormone ban in 2004, this led numerous supplement companies to pursue 'ephedra-free' formulations; many of which contain ingredients that have either been deemed by some health professionals as potentially harmful or haven't been researched for safety and effectiveness altogether. Prominent examples of controversial and/or obscure ingredients present in thermogenic products include (but are not limited to):

- Synephrine: adverse events have been linked to this ingredient (i.e., stroke in two healthy men, a heart attack in a previously healthy man taking Nutrex's Lipo-6x™, and ventricular fibrillation in an otherwise healthy military women as examples) and it has been deemed particularly harmful to persons predisposed to cardiovascular events

- Hordenine: present in numerous weight-loss supplements; it has been shown to stimulate catecholamine secretion which is theoretically as harmful to persons predisposed to cardiovascular events; more research is needed to confirm safety for human consumption

- Amine-based compounds (1,3-dimenthylamine, phenethylamine, methoxyphenylethylamine present in MHP's Dren™ weight loss product): these ingredients are commonly found in numerous weight-loss supplements; no research has evaluated this ingredient's efficacy or safety with long-term use

- Thyroid-mimetics (i.e., guggulsterones, 3,5 diiodo-l-thyronine as examples): evidence suggests that these compounds act to mimic thyroid hormones and may even confer positive health benefits in unhealthy rats; more research is needed to confirm safety for human consumption (i.e., lack of a hyperthyroid-like symptoms with use)

Recent media attention has also shed negative light on thermogenic supplements. In 2009, the FDA warned consumers to stop purchasing Iovate's old formulation of Hydroxycut, based upon 23 anecdotal reports of liver-related complications possibly linked with the use of Hydroxycut. In response to these issues, Iovate removed the old formula from the market and developed a new formula that is currently sold. The attribution of these health problems to the use of Hydroxycut has been debated, especially given that Iovate is considered to be one of the largest funders of supplement research and product safety on the market. Nonetheless, this example reinforces the notion that negative side effects can potentially occur in response to nutritional supplements on a person-to-person basis. In this regard, Dr. Jarret Morrow maintains an internet column (http://www.jarretmorrow.com) that reviews sports supplements. In an online column reviewing thermogenic beverages, he warned consumers that *"With the increasing popularity of energy drinks, it's important to be cognizant of the potential adverse effects associated with their consumption. Cases of seizures have been reported, Psychiatric sequelae have been reported by patients with known psychiatric illness, cardiovascular side effects* [including] *increased heart rate, blood pressure, cardiac arrest, and supraventricular tachycardia* [and] *stroke* [have also been reported]." Therefore, the consumer must: a) be aware of everything that is in the product that he/she consumes, and b) a personal predisposition to undesirable effects can be experienced.

Conclusions

It is ultimately up to athletes and fitness enthusiasts alike (as well as parents of children who partake in sports supplements) to be completely aware of what he/she is consuming on a day to day basis. As part of the *"Nutritional and Physical Performance: A Century of Progress and Tribute to the Modern Olympic Movement"* symposium given at a scientific meeting, lecturer Louis Grivetti detailed the innovative practices of the Greek philosopher Pythagoras of Samos (580-500 B.C.) who is considered the first person to train athletes on a high-meat diet. Pythagoras clearly recognized the need for nutritional adequacy to support the demands of rigorous training and his practices have led to the arrival of scientifically-based nutritional supplementation practices that have positively advanced athletic competition. However, , it is advised that patrons vigilantly research each ingredient on the back of supplement bottles prior to purchasing products. It is also advised that people avoid the non-medical use of anabolic steroids for the aforementioned health reasons. For athletes, the World Anti Doping Agency (WADA, http://www.wada-ama.org/) provides an annual online list of banned substances that have been adopted by hundreds of international sports organizations. This list is in a PDF format and has a convenient search tool for athletes, parents, or coaches to search for substances that are banned from competition. It is also preferable that novice consumers seek advice from his/her physician, nutritionist and coach prior to undertaking a nutritional supplement regimen. Dr. Richard Kreider and other renowned sports nutrition researchers have also published the "International Society Sports Nutrition Exercise & Sport Nutrition Review on Research & Recommendations" which provides consumers numerous guidelines as to how to assess the efficacy and safety of over-the-counter supplements. Finally, consumers are advised to access PubMed which archives scientific studies that outline the efficacy and safety of dietary supplement ingredients (http://www.ncbi.nlm.nih.gov/pubmed/). Extreme caution should be exercised in consuming supplements containing ingredients that have not been scientifically tested in animals and (preferably) humans. An important perspective to keep is that nutritional supplements should be viewed as a supplement to (and not substitute for) a lifestyle centered around regular exercise and healthy eating.

CHAPTER 9
Effective Training Methods to Build Strength:
Eliminating the need for Steroids and Hormones

So many of today's athletes have adopted the physical version of the "Get Rich Quick" scheme; instead of investing time, effort, and planning into their physical development, most athletes today would rather spend their energy on trying to uncover the quickest & easiest tactics for building the most trivial of gains in performance. Thanks to multi-million dollar advertising campaigns, the internet, and the arrival of new extreme sports into the mainstream media, every teenager to young adult now believes that they can be the next 'ultimate fighter' or professional ball player just by using some new piece of equipment or fancy supplement for a few days. Substances like stimulants and Nitric Oxide stimulators are just a few of the alleged 'necessities' needed for making 'real' gains in athleticism nowadays. Never before have there been so much false advertisements, propaganda tactics, and unsubstantiated material that, with the use of the media and internet, are so easily delivered directly to the eyes and ears of young athletes.

The aim of the following contribution will be to provide the reader with a set of principles and shared experiences that will eliminate the need for any "Get Better Quick" shortcuts. Any trainee will be able to use this blue print as a basis for achieving safe, sustainable, and transferrable gains in performance. In this chapter and in chapter 10, we will look at developing the two primary building blocks that must be in place if athletic performance is to be elevated: Strength & Endurance.

Building the foundation

In any training program, the first question that must be asked is, "What is the experience level or training age of the trainee?" The term 'training age' must be defined. For me and in the context of this book, training age is *the amount of time an individual has consistently trained under a **qualified coach**.* 'Training age' can be loosely defined and fabricated by anyone going through what they call 'workouts'. It amazes me every summer when the new signees arrive to begin their strength program, that ALL of them came from 'the best high school strength program in the country!' This reigns true until we get inside the weight room. What we see is as much a sure thing as the sun rising in the morning; 3/4s of the group cannot bodyweight squat properly, ½ can't hold an isometric lunge for more than 20 seconds, the other ½ can't perform a proper push up, and only 3 or 4 kids out of 20 can perform 5 real pull ups. Athletic position and technically sound movement are completely unfamiliar to them!

It is a principle of ours to start with the basics, and if you are a newcomer your training age is Zero. There are a small percentage of newcomers that do come from quality high school strength programs and have a basic understanding of how to work hard, but either way they have never trained under *us*. Therefore, in our system, with our test protocols, technical variances, team goals, and program progressions, every new athlete starts at the bottom and works their way up through the more advanced methods of building strength. It is my recommendation to any person looking to embark on a training program that they do the same; Start with the basics.

A few general principles of importance will be outlined and should be adhered to when taking part in strength training:

- Longevity is the <u>top priority</u> in a good Strength Training Program

- The main outcome being pursued by any trainee is the ability to perform on their playing field at a higher level. In order to do this, the athlete must first STAY on the playing field; injury prevention is the driving force behind all strength training & conditioning. It doesn't make any sense to be held back on the playing field due to inappropriate stresses endured throughout the off-season. Strength Training should be directed or prescribed by an experienced professional to avoid falling victim to any unwarranted methods that could slow down or counteract athletic development.

- A proper warm up or preparation period should always precede a training session.

- Core body temperature, heart rate, and alertness should all be elevated prior to training to ensure that the risk of injury is lessened. Also, it is important to understand that certain body regions and systems need to be excited and/or activated before they can function efficiently. 10-15 minutes of dynamic mobility and joint mobilization work should be done prior to the start of any performance training. It is also a good idea to undergo a bit of stabilization work during this period for those joints that require it; the knee, lumbar spine (or 'Core') and scapula (or Posterior Shoulder).

- Mobility drills should be trained in multiple planes in order to activate and innervate all muscles that move a joint. Joints that require sufficient mobility are the ankle, hip and thoracic spine.

- An optional beneficial addition to the beginning part of any warm up is myofascial release; these techniques will improve tissue quality and break up any tension in fatigued muscle. Foam Rollers, and other various forms of self serving modalities can be purchased for reasonable prices today.

- Free weights and body weight movements will almost always trump the use of machines.

- Machines operate on a fixed axis of movement, and the training residuals gained from their implementation do not translate well into the athletic realm. Sport is chaotic. If the body is conditioned to function in a rigid, un-chaotic fashion (like it will be if machines are primarily utilized), injuries are sure to come. Since machines do not permit movements that can rely heavily on synergistic stabilization across multiple joints, the major needs for sport preparation will not be met.

- Bodyweight movements like Push Ups, Pull Ups and Single Leg Squats/Step Ups, etc. provide the benefits of heightened body control, improved relative strength and functional capacity at the major joints and surrounding musculature.

- Machines aren't always bad. If an athlete is recovering from an injury, or in cases of disability, the use of a machine can provide the necessary stimulus to strengthen key musculature. Also, if an athlete has just completed a very demanding period of the year (12 straight weeks of off-season training), or is in the middle of an in-season phase, training with machines can be a beneficial change of pace on the body. The lower stress level that is inherent with the use of machines can allow for greater physical regeneration and recovery while maintaining the strength of skeletal muscle.

- Regardless of the reasoning for their inclusion, machine training should always be used in a limited and very strategic fashion.

- The majority of movements that make up the training program should aim to involve the maximal amount of muscles, over the most joints.

- In regards to exercises, size matters. The bigger the movement, or perhaps more clearly, the more joints required to complete the movement, equate to the more musculature being trained. This is another way of saying, "Bigger movements give you more return on your investment," and that is always a good thing when training for the type of strength required for athletic competition.

- This is another pitfall of working with machines. Most machines are based on the movement of a single joint. When thinking about an athlete's preparation, it is important that we always act in a manner that somewhat simulates the environment the athlete plays in. Most sports are played with athletes having their two feet on the ground. Very few machines allow the trainee to stand while working. A term like 'sport specific training' gets thrown around a lot, and misconceived even more. Within the confines of this book, we will define sport specific training as: athletic based training that stresses the body's systems in the same general, fundamental manner as the respective sport. *General, fundamental manner* for most sports includes: movement through multiple planes, ground based activity, transfer of power from the ground up through the body, starting & stopping, changing direction while moving explosively, and specific endurance, to name a few.

- Train for movement before muscle, but understand that you can't train one without the other.

- One of the first things to do is evaluate an athlete's ability to perform the most basic of bodyweight movements: Push Up, Pull Up/Chin Up, Inverted Row, Double Leg Squat, RDL/Good-morning, Lunge/Split Squat, Plank and Side Plank are great starting points for a sound strength training program. Evaluating these positions can either be from a visual screen or isometric holds for set amounts of time. If a position cannot be held for at least 30 seconds, the individual should work at strengthening the isometric capacity of the involved muscles before loading the movement pattern with external resistance. 30 seconds is a good starting point, and 60 seconds is a good goal to progress towards. After an athlete attains the conditioning needed to maintain a position for 60 seconds at the required range of motion, you can rest assured that they are ready for external loading.

__Isometric Split Squat__   __Isometric Side Plank__   __Isometric Squat Hold__

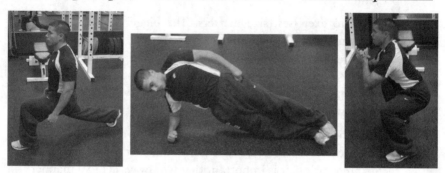

- Only after the key body positions have been learned and trained, are movements ready to be loaded. If this process is rushed, the athlete would simply be adding insult to injury by further ingraining improper and inefficient movement patterns. There is no quicker and more certain path to inviting injury. To foreshadow the importance of a topic I will touch on later; the initial loading of a beginning athlete should be always be manageable and progress to heavier over due time.

- If, or more appropriately *when*, these important body positions cannot be reached, there is usually a deficiency in place in the functional anatomy of the athlete. In cases like this, more work in the form of dynamic mobility, joint stabilization and/or corrective exercise is required.

- If you've developed the "Mirror Mentality," it's time to un-learn it.

- Because we can see our chest, shoulders, and abdominals in the mirror, we tend to worry about those muscle groups the most. Real athletic power will come from musculature that you cannot see in the mirror; your back, glutes and hamstrings. We have to develop an affinity for the muscles on the back side of our body if we are to improve our performance.

- What's the first exercise you learned? THE BENCH PRESS! Chances are you've been working towards a bigger bench for some time now. While the Bench Press is a good upper body strength builder, it's not the best choice for building an athletically durable, powerful body. If injury prevention and better body control are your goals, you will have to starting pulling and rowing more than you are pressing. Too much pressing in relation to pulling can lead to several problems ranging from reduced mobility in the upper body, painful shoulder impingement and rotator cuff problems. Protect your body by adding at least as many, if not more sets of exercises that involve pulling or rowing rather than pressing.

- Building strength one leg at a time is absolutely critical for developing athleticism.

- Most sports involve a great amount of running, jumping, cutting and landing on one leg in various positions and speeds at times throughout competition and practice. If sport requires the single leg to be the primary vehicle of movement for the duration of activity, wouldn't it be smart to develop lower body strength in that same manner? Sticking to the principles we have already discussed, some of the best single leg movements to use are:

- Barbell Step Up
- Dumbbell Lunge
- Front Squat Position Reverse Lunge
- Rear Foot Elevated Goblet Split Squat

Front Squat Position   **_Reverse Lunge_**

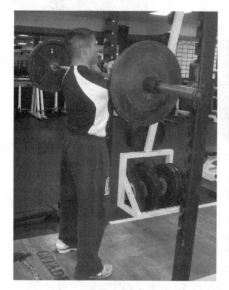 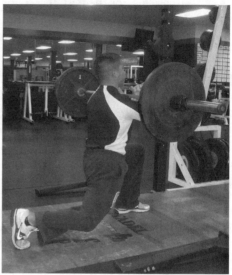

Rear Foot Elevated (RFE)   **_Goblet Split Squat_**

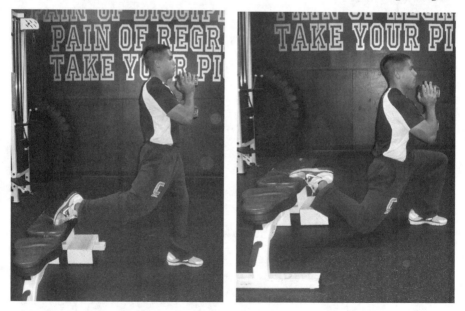

- There is a considerable amount of balance and coordination involved with single leg movements that will carry over to the field as well. Many injuries that occur in competitive sports are the result of a stabilizing muscle being too under-conditioned to maintain a respective joint's integrity while placed in an at-risk, unfamiliar position. In these situations, the load will either be compensated for by a nearby, less capable muscle, or the involved tissue will be injured. These undesired outcomes are preventable by strengthening and reinforcing the very stabilizing musculature that is inherently trained as an aspect of single leg training.

- Progression is the key to avoiding plateaus.

- All exercise progressions should follow a 'simple to complex' flow. If we make sure to start with the basics, working up to the more advanced or complicated methods will be feasible. If progressions are skipped and the continuum is too quickly moved through, strength gains will not be maintained and training residuals will be difficult to apply to sport.

An Example of a Lower Body Exercise Progression

Simple	⟶		Complex
Isometric Split Squat	Split Squat	DB Split Squat	Split Squat Jump

- In terms of building strength, 'Progression' is synonymous with 'Variation.' The human body is nothing more than an adaptive organism, and like all adaptive organisms its chief function is to respond to stimuli. Many people stick to a plan for years without seeing any real strength gains after their first 2-3 years. If stagnation occurs, you can rest assured that your body has stopped responding to the stimuli! Change in the form of introducing new movements is the no brainer, but sometimes you can get away with an even more subtle approach. Simply changing the angle of a joint, range of motion through a lift, type of implement, or tempo being used can shock a stale body and cause it to begin the adaptive process again.

- Progressions can also be helpful when preparing for different phases of the training year. If the off-season progresses from basic to complex, or moderately stressful to extremely stressful, would it make sense to progress into INSANELY stressful training during the pre/in-season?! NO! This would be a situation where progressing backwards would help maintain a healthy athlete. Progressions can get both harder and easier, and should, depending on where a trainee is in the training year.

- Strength training should also follow a course based on the strength-speed continuum; true explosive power & speed cannot be achieved without establishing baseline (foundation) strength first.

Priority	Strength – Speed Continuum	Examples
Priority #4	REACTIVE STRENGTH	Training that occurs in open space, involving movements done at maximum velocity, changes of direction & sustained effort over short durations. (speed, agility & quickness drills performed in 10 seconds or less)
Priority #3	EXPLOSIVE STRENGTH	Externally loaded movements done under high velocity (Olympic lifts, medicine ball throws, seated jumps, explosive traditional lifts with lighter loads and for fewer repetitions)
Priority #2	ABSOLUTE STRENGTH	Externally loaded movements done under control & under high muscle tension (traditional lifts: Squat, Bench, Deadlift)
Priority #1	RELATIVE STRENGTH	Movements or positions that create tension on muscles where the body is the only load present.(Bodyweight exercises, isometric holds, core training, dynamic mobility, eccentric movements)

It is important to understand that while the priorities have been labeled #1 – 4, this is not meant to show a ranking. Priority #4 could in fact be considered the most important one on the list; mastering this level and reaping its benefits will best help the athlete approach mastery in their sport (so long as it is a sport that requires movement in open space). The Priorities are assigned numbers to alert the trainee that they should focus on each Priority in numerical order first, and master each one before moving on to the next. Without mastering a specific Priority, training under the modalities in the next numerical level would be ill-advised; the training residuals of the later Priority will not be fully attainable until the residuals from the previous level have been realized and acquired.

- Olympic Lifts & Non-traditional methods of strength training can be a great progression added in to the later phases of a program.
- The Olympic Lifts are the Clean & Jerk and Snatch. Each lift can be broken down into several phases or variations. There are many advocates of the Olympic Lifts being included in training programs. Like any exercise, these lifts have pros and cons. Regardless of their benefits, the Olympic Lifts and all their variations should be utilized in a strategic way that seeks to capitalize on their results. Also, they should only be installed when a trainee has developed a solid strength base, good coordination, and an understanding of complex movements.

Pros & Cons of the Olympic Lifts

Pros	Cons
*Great amount of musculature involved	*Large learning curve – more instruction required
*Rate of force development = very high	*Olympic Lifts are a sport in themselves: carry over may be relatively low to respective playing fields
*High level of balance & coordination involved	
*High Nervous System involvement	*In large groups, difficult to properly supervise due to their high velocity of movement

- Implements like kegs, Atlas Stones, Medicine Balls, Kettlebells, thick ropes, heavy chain, tractor tires and sandbags can be a challenging addition to any training regimen. With these odd shaped implements, instability comes into play, and difficulty of movement is increased making it possible to evoke new adaptations from the body. Another up side to non-traditional training is that many of these types of objects allow for loaded 'every day' movements. An example would be doing walking lunges with a 100lb sandbag on one of your shoulders; the free forming shape of the bag would allow it to rest on one side of the body, causing a need for heightened stabilization in the torso.
- There is a fun-factor that comes with this type of training. Non-traditional means can be a great way to break up the monotony of a long, consistent program. They can also serve as superb ways to

end a training session. Many of the above named implements can be used in different types of competitions or medleys that can be as enjoyable as they are demanding.

- Non-traditional methods are NOT for beginners. They should be limited to 1-2 days per week maximum and used in a closely monitored environment. Even a moderate amount of overexposure to these types of exercises can carry with it a high risk of injury in an unprepared trainee. Only introduce Non-traditional means after at least 6-10 weeks of consistent traditional strength training. An exception is the Medicine Ball; due to the low risk of injury associated with the basic throws, Medicine Balls can be an excellent method for teaching athletes how to explosively unload effort into an implement.

- Building strength is like building anything worthwhile: it takes planning, dedication, and effort.

- Milo of Croton was an Olympian from ancient Greece. He is storied as one of the strongest and greatest Olympians of his time. His story begins when he, as a young boy, would carry his pet calf across his plot of land. As time went on, Milo continued to perform the feat as a show of strength to onlookers. Soon, the calf became a cow, and Milo a man. Since he had continued the task for so long, even as the animal got much bigger, Milo was able to carry on. This is one of the oldest stories that highlight what is now known as 'progressive overload.' The key to progressive overload is consistency over time. A trainee must train at certain lifts and gradually increase the load as time goes on; this is how the body gets stimulated to grow & remodel itself.

- While loading and overloading are important, rest and recovery are just as important. The body does not grow while training; it grows while recovering from the stress of previous training sessions. Planning periods of 'downloading' or 'unloading' is crucial to the success of all strength training programs. If the body is not given time for it to catch up to the training, the physical response will not be optimal.

- One of the best pieces of advice in regards to training is, "Listen to your body." Your body will tell you when it is time to back off from loading. Every person's physical make up and rate of recovery will be different. What's mandatory for some will be unnecessary to others. Some people can get away with 8 weeks of progressive overload, while most will need more frequent drop offs to accommodate for safe recovery.

- The longer an athlete has adhered to a training program, the more important the back off weeks will become, especially if we are to take into account variables like school, work, practice, etc. Three months of consistent training is adequate time to make considerable gains in strength before need to take a week or two off.

- When speaking about consecutive weeks of training, a good rule of thumb is "3 up, 1 down." This is in regard to the number of weeks devoted to loading. In any four week period of training, it is a good idea to 'back off' of the loading for at least 1 week. The cycle might look like one of these options:

Basic Loading Cycle – Option A

Week 1	Week 2	Week 3	Week 4
Moderate	*Hard*	*Maximal*	*Easy*
INTRO	LOAD	TEST	UNLOAD
4 sets / 6 reps each	*5 sets / 5 reps each*	*6 sets / 3-5 reps each*	*4 sets / 4 reps each*
* trainee should learn movements with light to moderate loads * No failure is permitted on this week	* load is increased to be slightly more difficult than previous week * Failure is still avoided here: once the movement is learned, load should be increased very gradually	* load will increase here until trainee can not overcome it * training needs to be closeley monitored and stopped once technical failure is reached * plenty of rest is needed in between sets (2-3 minutes)	* the weight is brought down to allow for recovery on this week * difficulty of sets should be lower than the INTRO week

Basic Loading Cycle – Option B

Week 1 *Moderate*	**Week 2** *Hard*	**Week 3** *Easy*	**Week 4** *Maximal*
INTRO	LOAD	UNLOAD	TEST
4 sets / 6 reps each	*5 sets / 5 reps each*	*4 sets / 4 reps each*	*6 sets / 3-5 reps each*
* trainee should learn movements with light to moderate loads * No failure is permitted on this week	* load is increased to be slightly more difficult than previous week * Failure is still avoided here: once the movement is learned, load should be increased very gradually	* the weight is brought down to allow for recovery on this week * difficulty of sets should be lower than the INTRO week	* load will increase here until trainee can not overcome it * training needs to be closeley monitored and stopped once technical failure is reached * plenty of rest is needed in between sets (2-3 minutes)

Beginning a Program

Using the foundational principles outlined above, you will be able to make effective progress from here on out in your training. There are different ways to split your training plan up; total body training sessions vs. body region split. We have found that for the average trainee, a 4 day per week, upper/lower split program tends to be the most effective. The more experienced a lifter becomes, the need for more complex and strategic planning is needed. But, this does not become a major issue until training has been consistently abided by for 5-6 years. In my personal experience, even if an athlete comes from a great high school strength program, in which he has undergone 4 straight years of consistently sound training, the need for advanced methods is very limited. *Some* 4th & 5th year players at the collegiate level will need special attention to their programming, if the goal is to lift heavier weight. In the end, we are talking about a very small population; maybe 10% of the athletes on a team. For the other 90%, the 4 day split I will outline will prove sufficient enough to elicit the gains in strength needed to enhance performance.

The weekly routine will follow a general layout of UPPER, LOWER,

UPPER, LOWER, with an off day coming at the middle of the week. This format can really accommodate an athlete's imposed demands at practice and other outside variables like a job or academics. Periods of the year there are no sport practice or competitions are ideal for this training plan (off-season phases).

The training week would look like this:

Off-season Training Week

SUN	MON	TUES	WED	THURS	FRI	SAT
Off	Upper Body	Lower Body	Off	Upper Body	Lower Body	Off
	60 mins.	60 mins.		60 mins.	60 mins.	

Another benefit of this layout is the amount of rest between training emphases. There are 48 hours minimum between each successive Upper or Lower session. On the weekends, the trainee would have 72 hours of recovery before training the Lower body again. This is of great importance since type of lifting done during the off-season periods should be the most demanding of the year. Lastly, focusing on the upper or lower half of the body allows for relatively short training sessions (60 minutes). The ability to keep the individual sessions short will allow for greater physiological response to the training; long, marathon sessions will only deplete an athlete's energy stores and negatively impact their development as well as the other commitments in their lives.

Since there are 2 training sessions each week devoted towards the major body regions, exercise selection or loading parameters will need to be different on each day. This choice can change from cycle to cycle, but it is of a high priority that the same exact session does not be repeated in a given week. This will optimize adaptation in response to the training.

A sample off-season training cycle might look like this:

Off-season Training Program

Day 1	Day 2	Day 3	Day 4
Upper Body 1	*Lower Body 1*	*Upper Body 2*	*Lower Body 2*
1a) Bench Press x10,8,6,4	1a) DB Walking Lunge 3x6e	1a) DB Incline Bench 3x8-10	1a) Front Squat x10,8,6,4
1b) Inverted Row 3x8-10	1b) Barbell RDL 3x8	1b) Bent Barbell Row x10,8,6	1b) DB 1 leg Dead Lift 3x3e
2a) DB Lat. Shldr. Raise 3x8	2a) Overhand Pull Up x10,8,6	2a) DB Front Raise 3x8	2a) Underhand Pull Up 3x10
2b) DB Curl 3x10-12	2b) DB Goblet Squat 3x10-12	2b) E-Z Bar Curl 3x10-12	2b) DB Step Up 3x6e
2c) Back Extension 3x15	2c) Glute Ham Raise 3x6-8	2c) 45 Deg. Back Ext. 3x15	2c) Partner Glute Ham 3x6-8
3a) Overhead Press 3x6	3a) MB Chops 3x10	3a) DB 1 arm OH Press 3x6e	3a) MB Hip Toss 3x8e
3b) Dips 3x10-12	3b) Russian Twist 3x15e	3b) Diamond Push Up 3x15	3b) Supine Leg Raise 3x12-15
3c) Wrist Roller 3x3	3c) Hanging Knee Up 3x8-12	3c) Squeeze Gripper 3x6e	3c) Hanging Knee Circle 3x6e
4a) Strict Push Up 3xMAX **4b) Side Plank Hold 2x :45e**	4a) Post Stretch – Hams, Groin, Calves, Hip Flexors, Glutes, Quads	4a) Explosive Push Up 3x6-8 4b) Ab Wheel Rollouts 3x8	4a) Post Stretch – Hams, Groin, Calves, Hip Flexors, Glutes, Quads

*10-15 minutes of myofascial release, dynamic mobility, activation, and flexibility work should start all sessions.
*Supersets: perform A,B,C then rest before starting A again. Unless a conditioning effect is desired, pace should be medium.
*On all Supersets, rest should be adequate enough to permit full recovery before starting next round (usually 1 – 2 minutes).
*Weights should ALWAYS be recorded. Athletes will need to reference previous performances in order to set benchmarks.

There are certain times in an athlete's annual plan that would call for a lower frequency of training. During the off-season, 4 days of training each week would be necessary. However, once the competitive season is approached, the amount of time inside the weight needs to be lessened. Once pre-season starts, 2 days of training per week should be the amount of time devoted towards maintain strength gains and reducing injuries with resistance training. It is during this phase that the split should also be altered; since only 2 days of training will be conducted, a more effective plan would be to shift to total body training sessions. In this capacity, the athlete will address all major areas of the body twice each week. An upper/lower split at this point in the year would only allow for the major body regions to get trained once in a 7 day period. That is not enough exposure to maintain physical preparedness. Another important aspect of in-season training is to make sure any heavy or strenuous weight training is not done the day before, or day of any games. If training is necessitated the day before a game because of multiple competitions in the week, loads should be kept very manageable. The number of movements should be held to 5-8 with adequate rest intervals in between (1-2 minutes). The volume on these exercises should also be relatively low (i.e. 3-4 sets of 1-6 repetitions each). In a session like this, the focal points would be dynamic flexibility, joint stabilization, active recovery and moderate nervous system stimulation. Typically, day-before-game lifts are labeled "Regeneration" sessions (**Regen.**). Finally, training session time should be cut in a multi-competition sport's week; 45 minutes is a sufficient amount of time to train when playing 2-3 games in a single week. In-season training weeks should resemble the following:

In-season Training Week - 1 game in a week

SUN	MON	TUES	WED	THURS	FRI	SAT
Off	**Total Body/** Practice 60 mins.	Practice	**Total Body/** Practice 60 mins.	Practice	Practice	**Competition**

In-season Training Week - 2 games in a week

SUN	MON	TUES	WED	THURS	FRI	SAT
Off	**Total Body/** Practice 45 mins.	Practice	**Competition**	**Total Body/** Practice 45 mins.	Practice	**Competition**

In-season Training Week - 3 games in a week

SUN	MON	TUES	WED	THURS	FRI	SAT
Off	Competition	Total Body/ Practice	Practice	Competition	Regen./ Practice	Competition
		45 mins.			45 mins.	

A sound in-season program for a sport that plays one game per week would resemble the following:

In-season Training Program

Day 1	Day 2
Total Body 1	***Total Body 2***
1a) DB Bench Press 4x5 1b) Isometric Plank Hold 3x :45 1c) Cross Over Step Up 3x5e	1a) Barbell Incline Press x6,5,4,3 1b) Isometric Side Plank Hold 3x :45 1c) RFE 1DB Goblet Split Squat 3x5e
2a) DB Lateral Shoulder Raise 3x8 2b) Underhand Pull Up 4x5 2c) Plate Back Extension 25# 3x10 2d) Band Groin Adduction 3x8e	2a) Side Lying Shoulder External Rotation 3x8e 2b) Standing 1 arm Cable Pull Down 3x8e 2c) 1 leg Reverse Hyper Extension 3x8e 2d) Slide Board Lateral Lunge 3x5e

10-15 minutes of myofascial release, dynamic mobility, activation, and flexibility work should start all sessions.
Movement on all exercises should be strict & controlled. Any bouncing should be deliberately avoided.
Supersets: perform A,B,C then rest before starting A again. Unless a conditioning effect is desired, pace should be medium.
On all Supersets, rest should be adequate enough to permit full recovery before starting next round (usually 1 – 2 minutes).
Weights should ALWAYS be recorded. Athletes will need to reference previous performances in order to set benchmarks.

Once the In-season phase is completed, there should be a period of active recovery that lasts for 2-4 weeks minimum, where no heavy lifting is done. During this time, activity should be limited to very non-intensive, sporadic sessions. The body will need to recover from any injuries sustained during the season, and the athlete needs this down time for energy levels to fully replenish. If this period is overlooked, an athlete can run the risk of overtraining which will extremely slow down their progress leading up to the next season. Once the body is fully recovered, and the athlete feels revitalized, training in the off-season should commence once again.

CHAPTER 10
Effective Training Methods to Build Endurance: Eliminating the need for Stimulants

The term 'endurance' can be misleading, and is often used loosely to describe the ability to run for long durations. Endurance is not specific to running. It is an aspect of athleticism that is critical for an athlete to be successful in any sport. Over the years, the term 'endurance' has become synonymous with 'cardiovascular conditioning,' or 'aerobic training.' This misconception has had a negative impact on athletes looking to improve their performance. In the following pages, we will discuss effective ways of improving real endurance that will lead to a direct increase in sport performance. First, we will define the term endurance as it is related to team sports:

Endurance: an athlete's ability to maintain a high level performance over the course of a competition.

This is not the same thing as 'being able to exercise for long durations.' For whatever reason many years ago, people decided that the ability to continue activity for time was the sure fire way to build or predict endurance. This is why many sport coaches had their athletes run 2-5 miles for time and used that as the predictor of potential. We now know that an athlete who runs fast and explosively changes direction is much more likely to help a team win games than one that moves slower but can do so for a longer amount time. Even if the coaches of yester-year knew this, they might not have known how to develop attributes like speed, agility and power in a team setting. Such was the pickle they found themselves in: "We need a faster team, BUT we don't know how to build that quality, so what's the next best thing? Simple answer

– make them run for longer amounts of time because the more we 'get in shape' the better off we'll be." In his book, 'Advances in Functional Training,' Mike Boyle said "it's easier to demand volume & effort than for coaches to learn the finer points of speed and power development."

Endurance should be viewed as the body's ability to fuel muscle activity, fight fatigue and recover during games and practice. This is a critical factor in performance. If an athlete's endurance is weak, their potential to perform is also weak. Even non-athletes need to understand this concept; simply exercising for great lengths of time in order to 'stay in shape' is a very flawed plan of attack. Training should always be results oriented, and without a basic understanding of what adaptations will come from a training stimulus, there can be no concrete direction.

There are different kinds of endurance, and depending on your sport or training goal, some will be more important that the others. In any case, the development of endurance should lead towards some specific outcome. If the desired outcome is to excel at a team sport, then endurance becomes very specific and will need to be planned in a tactical manner in order to avoid injury and reach the desired destination.

This chapter will not be aimed at educating the athlete on the chemical functions that make up bioenergetics. Instead, I will target the material towards providing you with an applicable menu of endurance training means, and layout a year-long plan that will aid in competition preparation.

Just like on the strength side of things, the endurance world is filled with false claims of easy ways to reach achievement. Stimulants are one of the most common products pushed on consumers as a reliable supplement to aid in training. In fact, any stimulant would serve more of a risk than any positive benefit. Dehydration, high heart rate, muscle cramping and inability to focus are all side effects of stimulants. For any person in training these effects are invitations to major setbacks, primarily in the form of injuries. There are safe and effective methods of building specific endurance that can take your game to the next level, which we will now discuss.

A Brief Overview of the Body's Energy Systems

Muscle activity is fueled by one of three Energy Systems in the body. Without getting too scientifically in-depth, I will give you a very basic overview of their properties and functions so that you may begin to understand how endurance can be developed.

Biological Energy Systems (or Metabolic Pathways)

Metabolic Pathway	Also known as	Produces energy for	Typical Intensity of Movements	Rate of depletion
Alactic Anaerobic	Phospho-Creatine System	0-6 seconds	Very High	Fastest
Lactic Anaerobic	Glycolytic System	6-180 seconds	Moderate – High	Moderate
Aerobic	Oxidative System	> 180 seconds	Low - Moderate	Slowest

As you can see, each energy system has specific properties that make it more or less effective at fueling certain actions. It should be noted, that while each energy system is specifically responsible for its own respective types of activity, all three are inter-related. There is no strict cut-off point where one system ceases work, and the next turns on. Each energy system is utilized based on the intensity of movement required. An activity done for 2 seconds at maximal intensity will call upon the Alactic Anaerobic Pathway, while an intense activity done for 60 seconds will first trigger the Alactic Anaerobic followed by the Lactic Anaerobic Pathway after 6-10 seconds. Not all sports are over and done within a single bout. Most team sports are played over the course of hours, consisting of repeated movements and intermittent stops, which can be considered rest intervals. In plain English; if you're 'endurance' training is conditioning the wrong energy system, you will not acquire the ability to outlast or outperform your opponents. And, in some cases, you might even weaken some of the capabilities that made you effective in the first place; if an explosive athlete is conditioned in a predominantly slow environment, that athlete will take on the characteristics of a less explosive one and performance will fall off. This is precisely why endurance training must be specific to the needs of the athlete in order to improve.

Building Sport Specific Endurance

There are two sides to the endurance equation:

Bioenergetics	Athletic Preparedness
*Speed at which energy is produced	*Efficiency of energy usage (sport skill)
*Ability to supply substrates	*Exposure of body to imposed demands
*Ability to utilize energy	(intensity of movement, environment)
*Ability to clear wasteful byproducts of energy	*Familiarity of 'game speed'
*Duration energy can be produced for	

An athlete with great endurance will have a balance between these two sides, and understand when to focus on developing one more than the other (we will deal in this area shortly). The fuel of the vehicle (Bioenergetics) might be optimal, but if the body of the car (physical preparedness) is not ready for the demands of the road (sport), the trip is sure to be bumpy. True Sport Specific Endurance is not as simple as maintaining a healthy cardiovascular system; it has more to do with preparing the body to endure the rigors of competition and practice. If a soccer player has poor change of direction mechanics, his/her efficiency of energy usage will suffer. If a tennis player's only exposure to the game has been 'teaching pace' sessions, his/her ability to perform at 'game speed' will not be strong. Both of these shortcomings would have a direct negative effect on the athlete's sport endurance.

On the other side of the coin, if an athlete has not developed their energy systems to handle their sport demands, all the Athletic Preparedness in the world won't help. The body needs to be able to supply & utilize energy as well as clear waste products in order for activity to continue. The key to enhancing endurance is to know which energy systems are the primary contributors to the respective sport, and what activities can best raise the Athletic Preparedness of the athlete.

Raising Athletic Preparedness

This is a commonly overlooked facet of endurance training. It is extremely important to train for sound movement mechanics. Energy needs to be utilized as efficiently as possible. If movement mechanics or technical skill is poor, energy will be wasted on compensatory action. This will undoubtedly limit an athlete's potential to perform well into the later stages of a game.

This can be avoided by making movement training be a part of the training regimen all year long.

Environmental constraints have a massive impact on the human body. When possible, train in an environment that is similar to what you will play in on game day. Training for endurance late in the afternoon to avoid the summer heat will not prepare a team that competes in the mid-day heat during their Competitive season. Planned sessions under the same environmental conditionings should begin at least 3-5 weeks before the season begins to allow for acclimatization.

A great strategy for raising your level of Athletic Preparedness is to simulate the speed and work to rest intervals seen on game day. The training process is not complete until some sort of metabolic simulation of the sport is introduced. When devising a metabolic program, you must find some specific data that is relative to the sport being played. For football, the metabolic demands are as follows:

- *Average length of play: 4-6 seconds of all out effort*

- *Typical rest between plays: 20-40 seconds of time in the huddle (no constant movement)*

- *Typical # of plays per game: 60-70 plays*

- *Rests coming at intermittent times for timeouts, quarters, and half-time*

From this information, the following program could be devised:

Series 1	Series 2	Series 3	Series 4
1. Sprint 20 yd	1. Pedal 5 turn & sprint 10 yd	1. 45 degree angle cuts 20 yd	1. Pedal 5 turn & sprint 10 yd
2. Pro shuttle	2. Sprint 20 yd	2. Pedal 5 turn & sprint 10 yd	2. Sprint 20 yd
3. Sprint 10 yd	3. Pro shuttle	3. Sprint 20 yd	3. Pro shuttle
4. Pedal 5 turn & sprint 10 yd	4. Sprint 10 yd	4. Pro shuttle	4. Lateral shuffle 5 & back, twice
5. Lateral shuffle 15 yd	5. 45 degree angle cuts 20 yd	5. Sprint 10 yd	5. Lateral shuffle 15 yd
6. Up down & sprint 10 yd	6. Pedal 10 yd Sprint back 10 yd	6. Pedal 10 yd Sprint back 10 yd	6. Up down & sprint 10 yd
7. Vertical jump & sprint 20 yd	7. Up down & sprint 10 yd	7. Vertical jump & sprint 20 yd	7. 45 degree angle cuts 20 yd
8. 45 degree angle cuts 20 yd	8. Vertical jump & sprint 20 yd	8. Lateral shuffle 5 & back, twice	8. Sprint 10 yd
9. Pedal 10 yd sprint back 10 yd	9. Lateral shuffle 5 & back, twice	9. Lateral shuffle 15 yd	9. Pedal 10 yd Sprint back 10 yd
10. Lateral shuffle 5 & back, twice	10. Lateral Shuffle 15 yd	10. Up down & sprint 10 yd	10. Vertical jump & sprint 20 yd

There would be a variable rest in between each 'play' of 20-40 seconds (simulating the typical time spent in the huddle). In between 'series,' there would be a 2-3 minute rest, and this would be considered a 'water break.' After completing the 4 series, it would be up to the coach to repeat which ever series they choose. This would be done until the desired amount of snaps was completed (60-70 plays). The versatility that comes with metabolic conditioning is what makes it so effective. Virtually any drill, exercise or running pattern can be installed into the blue print and, as long as the time parameters are followed, you will have a new training session to challenge you.

Training for Endurance over the Off-season

For most team sports, interval work should be the primary focus of endurance training. Long, slow, distance running (LSD) should be limited in the training year, unless the sport being trained for is in-fact distance running. Only in the early periods of training should any type of LSD running be utilized. This type of training should only be used as a 'stepping stone' to more stressful methods, if better work capacity is needed at the time. If an athlete is preparing for distance running, 1-3 sessions per week of LSD could be installed. 30-90 minutes is the preferred duration, while keeping the heart rate in 120-150 beats per minute range. This training will improve cardiac output, increase vascular density and lead to a better supply of oxygen to the muscular system. As with all types of performance training, a sound warm up consisting of soft tissue work, activation and mobility work should be done before beginning the session.

Interval training should be the method of choice for most athletes because of the physical demands placed on the body that are not present in LSD running. In sport, athletes start, stop, cut, and explosively maneuver in and out of different positions while exerting a high amount of effort. Interval work, in the form of shuttles, tempo runs, cone drills, etc., more closely simulates the arenas that most athletes play in. Without this type of training, certain muscles in the body would be underdeveloped and very unfamiliar to the movements that will occur on the playing field; there will not be a good resistance to injuries. Lastly, when dealing with intervals, the heart rate will be kept in the aerobic training range while resting between reps and even for some time after cessation. Because of this aerobic effect from the training, intervals are clearly more time efficient than traditional methods that can occupy an hour or more.

After the season has been completed, athletes are advised to take some time off from scheduled training. Once this Active Recovery period (2-4 weeks) is over, training for endurance can begin. Even though the next competitive season is a good ways away, it would not be in the best interest of the athlete to remove endurance training from their program; there should be a base line level of physical conditioning maintained all year. This will keep the General Physical Preparedness of the athlete up and allow for greater training gains. At times, particularly in the weeks leading up to competition, the endurance level of the athlete will be of higher importance:

Phase:	Active Rest Phase	Developmental Phase	Competitive Phase
Description:	2-4 weeks following the season	Period of the year when NO sport practice/ games are being held. Can have more than 1 Developmental Phase (sports with multiple seasons)	Period of the year when the majority of the training is devoted to specific sport practice and skill development.
Preferred type of Endurance Training:	none	Tempo Runs of 40-110 yards, Shuttles of 50-300 yards (25 yd legs), Metabolic Simulation	Shuttles of 50-300 yards
Frequency:	0 sessions/ week	2-4 sessions/week (should progress to greater frequency as Competitive Phase approaches)	0-2 sessions/ week
Volume:		Tempo Runs x10-20 reps, Shuttles x750-1500 yards/session, Metabolic Simulation x60-70 reps	Shuttles x500-1000 yds/session

Frequency during the Competitive Phase is cut down due to the fact that daily exposure to full speed play will be possible during practice. If one day of endurance training is preferred, it is important to not overload the athletes with too much specific drilling. If they are doing specific drilling for multiple hours every day practice, what more could be achieved from adding in more? During the Competitive Phase, sometimes the level of endurance that was built over the Developmental period can be lost since the amount of time devoted to general conditioning is significantly reduced. It is for this very reason, that the non-specific means should be included, if any at all.

Below you will find an 8 week long Endurance Training Program that could be used in most team sports. The program will have 2 training days every week which should be separated by 48 hours minimum. For the most part, 1 day of each week will be devoted to straight line running, and 1 day will committed to running that includes changes of direction. Shuttles can be done with 25-50 yard legs, but it should be understood that there will be a noticeable difference in their level of difficulty depending on their distance. The 25 yard set up will have more line tags be a bit more demanding than the 50 yard version. It is a good idea to start the program on the 50 yard set up and progress into the 25 yard version.

The final area for discussion will be the tempo under which all of these endurance drills should be run. With Metabolics being the lone exception, no Endurance training is done at what could be considered actual 100% full speed. The pace for this type of interval work is more 75%-85% range. You may feel like you're moving at full speed because of the difficulty of the drills, but you'll actually be at a pace. The rest intervals that are placed on this training will not allow the body to completely replenish energy stores making actual max speed unattainable. Running at this pace, and under those rest intervals, is what makes the cardiovascular system work hard enough to elicit the desired responses with interval training. Metabolics are a different type of interval training, which are more focused on the development on Alactic Anaerobic Pathway. They are meant to simulate and familiarize the body with the movements seen in sport, so they should always be executed at full speed, and only after a proper progression has led up to their inclusion.

8 Week Endurance Training Program

	Week 1	Week 2	Week 3	Week 4	Week 5	Week 6	Week 7	Week 8
Day:	1	1	1	1	1	1	1	1
Drill:	100 yd Tempo	100 yd Tempo	100 yd Tempo	60 yd Sprint	60 yd Sprint	Metabolics	Metabolics	Metabolics
Time:	<:14-:16	<:14:16	<:14:16	<:08	<:08	:04-06	:04-06	:04-06
Rest:	:45	:45	:45	:30	:30	:20-:40	:20-:40	:20-:40
Reps:	10	12	14	15	20	40 plays	50 plays	60 plays
Total Yds:	1000	1200	1400	900	1200	n/a	n/a	n/a
Day:	2	2	2	2	2	2	2	2
Drill:	100 yd Shuttle	100 yd Shuttle	100 yd Shuttle	200 yd Shuttle	200 yd Shuttle	300 yd Shuttle	300 yd Shuttle	300 yd Shuttle
Time:	<:20	<:20	<:20	<:40	<:40	<:60	<:60	<:60
Rest:	:60	:60	:40	2:00	2:00	3:00	2:30	2:00
Reps:	6	8	10	6	8	4	5	5
Total Yds:	600 yds	800 yds	1000 yds	1200 yds	1600 yds	1200 yds	1500 yds	1500 yds
Wk Total:	1600 yds	2000	2400	2100	2800			

References

Chapter 2

Abcouwer SF. The effects of glutamine on immune cells. Nutrition. 2000;16(1):67-69.

Astrom RE, Feigh M, Pedersen BK. Persistent low-grade inflammation and regular exercise. Front Biosci (Schol Ed). 2010 Jan 1;2:96-105.

Avenell A. Symposium 4: Hot topics in parenteral nutrition Current evidence and ongoing trials on the use of glutamine in critically-ill patients and patients undergoing surgery. Proc Nutr Soc. 2009 Jun 3:1-8.

Briones AM, Touyz RM Moderate exercise decreases inflammation and oxidative stress in hypertension: but what are the mechanisms? Hypertension. 2009 Dec;54(6):1206-8. Epub 2009 Oct 19.

Brown G D, Gordon S; "Immune recognition. A new receptor for beta-glucans." Sir William Dunn School of Pathology, Nature Sep 2001, 6;413(6851):36-7.

Buchman AL. Glutamine: commercially essential or conditionally essential? A critical appraisal of the human data. Am J Clin Nutr. 2001;74(1):25-32.

Carrillo AE, Murphy RJ, Cheung SS. Vitamin C supplementation and salivary immune function following exercise-heat stress. Int J Sports Physiol Perform. 2008 Dec;3(4):516-30.

Carver JD. Dietary nucleotides: effects on the immune and gastrointestinal systems. Acta Paediatr Suppl. 1999 Aug;88(430):83-8.

Colbert LH, Visser M, Simonsick EM, Tracy RP, Newman AB, Kritchevsky SB, Pahor M, Taaffe DR, Brach J, Rubin S, Harris TB. Physical activity, exercise, and inflammatory markers in older adults: findings from the Health, Aging and Body Composition Study. J Am Geriatr Soc.2004 Jul;52(7):1098-104.

Davis JM, Murphy EA, Carmichael MD, Zielinski MR, Groschwitz CM,

Brown AS, Gangemi JD, Ghaffar A, Mayer EP. Curcumin effects on inflammation and performance recovery following eccentric exercise-induced muscle damage. Am J Physiol Regul Integr Comp Physiol. 2007 Jun;292(6):R2168-73. Epub 2007 Mar 1.

Davis, J.M., M.L. Kohut, L.H. Colbert, D.A. Jackson, A. Ghaffar, and E.P. Mayer (1997). Exercise, alveolar macrophage function, and susceptibility to respiratory infection. Journal of Applied Physiology 83:1461-1466.

Depner CM, Kirwan RD, Frederickson SJ, Miles MP Enhanced inflammation with high carbohydrate intake during recovery from eccentric exercise. Eur J Appl Physiol. 2010 Aug;109(6):1067-76. Epub 2010 Apr 3.

Edwards, K. M., Burns, V. E., Ring, C., & Carroll, D. (2006). Individual differences in the interleukin-6 response to maximal and submaximal exercise tasks. Journal of Sports Sciences, 2006, 24(8), 855 – 862.

Fahlman, M.M., & Engels, Heman-J. (2005) Mucosal IgA and URTI in American collegiate football players: A year longitudinal study. Medicine & Science In Sport & Exercise, 2005, 37(3), 374 – 380

Fatouros IG, Destouni A, Margonis K, Jamurtas AZ, Vrettou C, Kouretas D, Mastorakos G, Mitrakou A, Taxildaris K, Kanavakis E, Papassotiriou I. Cell-free plasma DNA as a novel marker of aseptic inflammation severity related to exercise overtraining. Clin Chem. 2006 Sep;52(9):1820-4. Epub 2006 Jul 13.

Friman, G., and N.G. Ilback (1998). Acute infection: metabolic responses, effects on performance, interaction with exercise, and myocarditis. International Journal of Sports Medicine 1998, 19(Suppl 3):S172-S182.

Ford ES. Does exercise reduce inflammation? Physical activity and C-reactive protein among U.S. adults. Epidemiology. 2002 Sep;13(5):561-8.

Gil A. Modulation of the immune response mediated by dietary nucleotides. Eur J Clin Nutr. 2002 Aug;56 Suppl 3:S1-4.

Gleeson, M. (2006). Can nutrition limit exercise-induced immunodepression? Nutrition reviews 2006, 64(3), 119 – 131.

Gleeson M, Exercise, nutrition and immune function. J Sports Sci. 2004 Jan;22(1):115-25.

Gleeson, M. Mucosal immunity and respiratory illness in elite athletes. International Journal of Sports Medicine, 2000, 21(1), S33 – S43.

Gleeson, M., A.K. Blannin, N.P. Walsh, N.C. Bishop, and A.M. Clark (1998). Effect of low- and high-carbohydrate diets on the plasma glutamine and circulating leukocyte responses to exercise. International Journal of Sport Nutrition 1998, 8:49-59.

Goussetis E, Spiropoulos A, Tsironi M, Skenderi K, Margeli A, Graphakos S, Baltopoulos P, Papassotiriou I. Spartathlon, a 246 kilometer foot race: effects of acute inflammation induced by prolonged exercise on circulating progenitor reparative cells. Blood Cells Mol Dis. 2009 May-Jun;42(3):294-9. Epub 2009 Feb 23.

Hunter KW, Gault RA, Berner MD, Preparation of microparticulate B-glucan from Saccharomyces cerevisiae for use in immune potentiation. Letters in Applied Microbiology, October 2002, Vol 35 Issue 4, 267-271,

Holen, E, Bjørge OA, Jonsson R.Dietary nucleotides and human immune cells. II. Modulation of PBMC growth and cytokine secretion. Nutrition. 2005 Oct;21(10):1003-9.

Jeurissen A, The effects of physical exercise on the immune system, Ned Tijdschr Geneeskd 2003 Jul 12;147(28):1347-51

Kelly GS. Nutritional and botanical interventions to assist with the adaptation to stress. Altern Med Rev. 1999 Aug;4(4):249-65.

Kim HJ, Lee YH, Kim CK. Biomarkers of muscle and cartilage damage and inflammation during a 200 km run. Eur J Appl Physiol. 2007 Mar;99(4):443-7. Epub 2007 Jan 6.

Kokkinos P. Exaggerated exercise blood pressure: is it all about inflammation? J Cardiopulm Rehabil. 2006 May-Jun;26(3):150-1.

Kogan G, Pajtinka M, Babincova M, Miadokova E, Rauko P, Slamenova D, Korolenko TA. Yeast cell wall polysaccharides as antioxidants and antimutagens: can they fight cancer? Neoplasma. 2008;55(5):387-93.

Konig, D., D. Grathwohl, C. Weinstock, H. Northoff, and A. Berg. Upper respiratory tract infection in athletes: influence of lifestyle, type of sport, training effort, and immunostimulant intake. Exercise Immunology Review 2000, 6:102-120.

Kulkarni AD, Rudolph FB, Van Buren CT. The role of dietary sources of nucleotides in immune function: a review. J Nutr. 1994 Aug;124(8 Suppl):1442S-1446S.

Maffulli, N., V. Testa, and G. Capasso. Post-viral fatigue syndrome. A longitudinal assessment in varsity athletes. Journal of Sports Medicine and Physical Fitness 1993, 33:392-399.

Matthews, C.E., I.S. Ockene, P.S. Freedson, M.C. Rosal, J.R. Herbert, and P.A. Merriam. Physical activity and risk of upper-respiratory tract infection. Medicine and Science in Sports and Exercise 2000, 32:S292. Nehlsen-Cannarella, S.L., D.C. Nieman, O.R. Fagoaga, W.J. Kelln, D.A.

Malm C. Exercise-induced muscle damage and inflammation: fact or fiction? Acta Physiol Scand. 2001 Mar;171(3):233-9.

Mc Naughton L, Bentley D, Koeppel P. The effects of a nucleotide supplement on the immune and metabolic response to short term, high intensity exercise performance in trained male subjects. J Sports Med Phys Fitness. 2007 Mar;47(1):112-8

Mc Naughton L, Bentley DJ, Koeppel P. The effects of a nucleotide supplement on salivary IgA and cortisol after moderate endurance exercise. J Sports Med Phys Fitness. 2006 Mar;46(1):84-9.

Monteleone, P, Beinat, L, Tanzillo,C, Maj, M, and Kemali, D. "Effects of phosphatidylserine on the neuroendocrine response to physical stress in humans." Neuroendocrinol, 1990. 52: 243-8.

Monteleone, P, Maj,M, Beinat,L, Natale,M, and Kemali,D. "Blunting by chronic phosphatidylserine administration of the stress-induced activation of the hypothalamos-pituitary-adrenal axis in healthy men." Eur. J. Clin.Pharmacol ,1992. 41: 385-8.

Nagafuchi S, Totsuka M, Hachimura S, Goto M, Takahashi T, Yajima T, Kuwata T, Kaminogawa S. Dietary nucleotides increase the proportion of a TCR gammadelta+ subset of intraepithelial lymphocytes (IEL) and IL-7 production by intestinal epithelial cells (IEC); implications for modification of cellular and molecular cross-talk between IEL and IEC by dietary nucleotides. Biosci Biotechnol Biochem. 2000 Jul;64(7):1459-6

Nakajima T, Kurano M, Hasegawa T, Takano H, Iida H, Yasuda T, Fukuda T, Madarame H, Uno K, Meguro K, Shiga T, Sagara M, Nagata T, Maemura K, Hirata Y, Yamasoba T, Nagai R. Pentraxin3 and high-sensitive C-reactive protein are independent inflammatory markers released during high-intensity exercise. Eur J Appl Physiol. 2010 Jul 17

Nieman, D. C., & Bishop, N. C. Nutritional strategies to counter stress to the immune system in athletes, with special reference to football. Journal of sports sciences 2006, 24(7), 763 – 772.

Nieman, D.C., S.L. Nehlsen-Cannarella, O.R. Fagoaga, D.A. Henson, A. Utter, J.M. Davis, F. Williams, and D.E. Butterworth. Influence of mode and carbohydrate on the cytokine response to heavy exertion. Medicine and Science in Sports and Exercise 1998, 30:671-678.

Nieman, D.C., S.L. Nehlsen-Cannarella, D.A. Henson, D.E. Butterworth, O.R. Fagoaga, and A. Utter. Influence of carbohydrate ingestion and mode on the granulocyte and monocyte response toheavy exertion in triathletes. Journal of Applied Physiology 1998, 84:1252- 1259.

Novak M, Vetvicka V. Glucans as biological response modifiers. Endocr Metab Immune Disord Drug Targets. 2009 Mar;9(1):67-75.

Novak M, Vetvicka V. Beta-glucans, history, and the present: immunomodulatory aspects and mechanisms of action. J Immunotoxicol. 2008 Jan;5(1):47-57.

Olsson EM, von Schéele B, Panossian AG.A randomised, double-blind, placebo-controlled, parallel-group study of the standardised extract shr-5 of the roots of Rhodiola rosea in the treatment of subjects with stress-related fatigue. Planta Med. 2009 Feb;

Acute Rhodiola rosea intake can improve endurance exercise performance. Int J Sport Nutr Exerc Metab. 2004 June7

Parsons JP, Baran CP, Phillips G, Jarjoura D, Kaeding C, Bringardner B, Wadley G, Marsh CB, Mastronarde JG. Airway inflammation in exercise-induced bronchospasm occurring in athletes without asthma. J Asthma. 2008 Jun;45(5):363-7.

Peake JM, Suzuki K, Coombes JS. The influence of antioxidant supplementation on markers of inflammation and the relationship to oxidative stress after exercise. J Nutr Biochem. 2007 Jun;18(6):357-71. Epub 2006 Dec 6.

Pedersen BK, Akerstrom TC, Nielsen AR, and Fischer CP, Role of myokines in exercise and metabolism, Journal of Applied Physiology, Mar 2007.

Peters EM, Anderson R, Nieman DC, Fickl H, Jogessar V. Vitamin C supplementation attenuates the increases in circulating cortisol, adrenaline and anti-inflammatory polypeptides following ultramarathon running. Int J Sports Med. 2001 Oct;22(7):537-43.

Peters EM, Anderson R, Theron AJ. Attenuation of increase in circulating cortisol and enhancement of the acute phase protein response in vitamin C-supplemented ultramarathoners. Int J Sports Med. 2001 Feb;22(2):120-6.

Rondanelli M, Opizzi A, Monteferrario F. The Biological activity of beta-glucans, Minerva Medical; Jun 2009 100(3):237-245;

Roubenoff R. Molecular basis of inflammation: relationships between catabolic cytokines, hormones, energy balance, and muscle. JPEN J Parenter Enteral Nutr. 2008 Nov-Dec;32(6):630-2.

Roubenoff R. Physical activity, inflammation, and muscle loss. Nutr Rev. 2007 Dec;65(12 Pt 2):S208-12.

Rudolph FB. Symposium: dietary nucleotides: a recently demonstrated requirement for cellular development and immune function. J Nutr. 1994 Aug;124(8 Suppl):1431S-1432S.

Sengupta K, Krishnaraju AV, Vishal AA, Mishra A, Trimurtulu G, Sarma KV, Raychaudhuri SK, Raychaudhuri SP. Comparative efficacy and tolerability of 5-Loxin and AflapinAgainst osteoarthritis of the knee: a double blind, randomized, placebo controlled clinical study. Int J Med Sci. 2010 Nov 1;7(6):366-77.

Sengupta K, Alluri KV, Satish AR, Mishra S, Golakoti T, Sarma KV, Dey D, Raychaudhuri SP.A double blind, randomized, placebo controlled study of the efficacy and safety of 5-Loxin for treatment of osteoarthritis of the knee. Arthritis Res Ther. 2008;10(4):R85.

Skarpanska-Stejnborn A, Pilaczynska-Szczesniak L, Basta P, Deskur-Smielecka The influence of supplementation with Rhodiola rosea L. extract on selected redox parameters in professional rowers. Int J Sport Nutr Exerc Metab. 2009 Apr;

Smith, L. L. Tissue trauma: The underlying cause of overtraining syndrome? Journal of strength and conditioning research 2004, 18(1), 185 – 193.

Spence, L., Brown, W. J., Pyne, D. B., Nissen, M. D., Sloots, T. P., McCormack, J. G., et al. Incidence, etiology, and symptomatology of upper respiratory illness in elite athletes. Medicine and science in sports and exercise 2007, 39(4), 577 – 586.

Stupka N, Lowther S, Chorneyko K, Bourgeois JM, Hogben C, Tarnopolsky MA. Gender differences in muscle inflammation after eccentric exercise. J Appl Physiol. 2000 Dec;89(6):2325-32.

Van Buren CT, Rudolph F. Dietary nucleotides: a conditional requirement. Nutrition. 1997 May;13(5):470-2.

Verde TJ, Immune responses and increased training of the elite athlete., J Appl Physiol. 1992 Oct;73(4):1494-9.

Vetvicka V, Vashishta A, Saraswat-Ohri S, Vetvickova J. Immunological effects of yeast- and mushroom-derived beta-glucans. J Med Food. 2008 Dec;11(4):615-22.

Woods JA, Vieira VJ, Keylock KT. Exercise, inflammation, and innate immunity. Immunol Allergy Clin North Am. 2009 May;29(2):381-93.

Chapter 3

Arent SM, Senso M, Golem DL, McKeever KH. The effects of theaflavin-enriched black tea extract on muscle soreness, oxidative stress, inflammation, and endocrine responses to acute anaerobic interval training: a randomized, double-blind, crossover study. J Int Soc Sports Nutr. 2010 Feb 23;7(1):11.

Banerjee AK, Mandal A, Chanda D, Chakraborti S. Oxidant, antioxidant and physical exercise. Mol Cell Biochem. 2003 Nov;253(1-2):307-12.

Bryant RJ, Ryder J, Martino P, et al.: Effects of vitamin E and C supplementation either alone or in combination on exerciseinduced lipid peroxidation in trained cyclists. J Strength Cond Res 2003, 17(4):792-800.

Bryer SC, Goldfarb AH. Effect of high dose vitamin C supplementation on muscle soreness, damage, function, and oxidative stress to eccentric exercise. Int J Sport Nutr Exerc Metab. 2006 Jun;16(3):270-80.

Carrera-Quintanar L, Funes L, Viudes E, Tur J, Micol V, Roche E, Pons A. Antioxidant effect of lemon verbena extracts in lymphocytes of university students performing aerobic training program. Scand J Med Sci Sports. 2010 Nov 18. [Epub ahead of print]

Childs A, Jacobs C, Kaminski T, et al.: Supplementation with vitamin C and N-Acetyl-Cysteine increases oxidative stress in humans after an acute muscle injury induced by eccentric exercise. Free Radical Biology & Medicine 2001, 31(6):745-753.

Clarkson PM, Thompson HS: Antioxidants: what role do they play in physical activity and health? Am J Clin Nutr 2000, 72(suppl):637S-646S.

Connolly DA, McHugh MP, Padilla-Zakour OI, Carlson L, Sayers SP: Efficacy of a tart cherry juice blend in preventing the symptoms of muscle damage. Br J Sports Med 2006, 40:679-83. Dekkers JC, van Doornen LJ, Kemper HC. The role of antioxidant vitamins and enzymes in the prevention of exercise-induced muscle damage. Sports Med. 1996 Mar;21(3):213-38

Fernández JM, Da Silva-Grigoletto ME, Gómez-Puerto JR, Viana-Montaner BH, Tasset-Cuevas I, Túnez I, López-Miranda J, Pérez-Jiménez F. A dose of fructose induces oxidative stress during endurance and strength exercise. J Sports Sci. 2009 Oct;27(12):1323-34.

Funes L, Carrera-Quintanar L, Cerdán-Calero M, Ferrer MD, Drobnic F, Pons A, Roche E, Micol V. Effect of lemon verbena supplementation on muscular damage markers, proinflammatory cytokines release and neutrophils' oxidative stress in chronic exercise. Eur J Appl Physiol. 2010 Oct 22. [Epub ahead of print]

Bloomer RJ, Goldfarb AH, McKenzie MJ, You T, Nguyen L. Effects of antioxidant therapy in women exposed to eccentric exercise. Int J Sport Nutr Exerc Metab. 2004 Aug;14(4):377-88.

Howatson G, McHugh MP, Hill JA, Brouner J, Jewell AP, van Someren KA, Shave RE, Howatson SA: Influence of tart cherry juice on indices of recovery following marathon running. Scand J Med Sci Sports 2009.

Kawada S, Kobayashi K, Ohtani M, Fukusaki C. Cystine and theanine supplementation restores high-intensity resistance exercise-induced attenuation of natural killer cell activity in well-trained men. J Strength Cond Res. 2010 Mar;24(3):846-51.

Kelly MK, Wicker RJ, Barstow TJ, Harms CA. Effects of N-acetylcysteine on respiratory muscle fatigue during heavy exercise. Respir Physiol Neurobiol. 2009 Jan 1;165(1):67-72. Epub 2008 Oct 17.

Kelley DS, Rasooly R, Jacob RA, Kader AA, Mackey BE: Consumption of bing sweet cherries lowers circulating concentrations of inflammation markers in healthy men and women. J Nutr 2006, 136:981-986.

Kerksick C, Willoughby D. The antioxidant role of glutathione and N-acetyl-cysteine supplements and exercise-induced oxidative stress. J Int Soc Sports Nutr. 2005 Dec 9;2:38-44.

Kuehl et al. REefsefairccha acrtiycl eof tart cherry juice in reducing muscle pain during running: a randomized controlled trial. Journal of the International Society of Sports Nutrition 2010, 7:17

Laaksonen DE, Atalay M, Niskanen L, Uusitupa M, Hänninen O, Sen CK. Blood glutathione homeostasis as a determinant of resting and exercise-induced oxidative stress in young men. Redox Rep. 1999;4(1-2):53-9.

Lee J, Clarkson PM: Plasma creatine kinase activity and glutathione after eccentric exercise. Med Sci Sports Exerc 2003, 35(6):930-936.

Margaritis I, Palazzetti S, Rousseau AS, Richard MJ, Favier A. Antioxidant supplementation and tapering exercise improve exercise-induced antioxidant response. J Am Coll Nutr. 2003 Apr;22(2):147-56.

Matuszczak Y, Farid M, Jones J, et al.: Effect of n-acetylcysteine on glutathione oxidation and fatigue during handgrip exercise. Muscle Nerve 2005, 32:633-638.

Medved I, Brown MJ, Bjorksten AR, et al.: N-acetylcysteine enhances muscle cysteine and glutathione availability and attenuates fatigue during prolonged exercise in endurance-trained individuals. J Appl Physiol 2004, 97:1477-1485.

Medved I, Brown MJ, Bjorksten AR, et al.: N-acetylcysteine infusion alters blood redox status but not time to fatigue during intense exercise in humans. J Appl Physiol 2003, 94:1572-1582.

Mickleborough TD, Lindley MR, Montgomery GS. Effect of fish oil-derived omega-3 polyunsaturated Fatty Acid supplementation on exercise-induced bronchoconstriction and immune function in athletes. Phys Sportsmed. 2008 Dec;36(1):11-7.

Mickleborough TD, Lindley MR, Ionescu AA, Fly AD. Protective effect of fish oil supplementation on exercise-induced bronchoconstriction in asthma. Chest. 2006 Jan;129(1):39-49.

Mickleborough TD, Murray RL, Ionescu AA, Lindley MR. Fish oil supplementation reduces severity of exercise-induced bronchoconstriction in elite athletes. Am J Respir Crit Care Med. 2003 Nov 15;168(10):1181-9. Epub 2003 Aug 6.

Naziroğlu M, Kilinç F, Uğuz AC, Celik O, Bal R, Butterworth PJ, Baydar ML. Oral vitamin C and E combination modulates blood lipid peroxidation and antioxidant vitamin levels in maximal exercising basketball players. Cell Biochem Funct. 2010 Jun;28(4):300-5.

Niess AM, Simon P. Response and adaptation of skeletal muscle to exercise--the role of reactive oxygen species. Front Biosci. 2007 Sep 1;12:4826-38.

Nikolaidis MG, Jamurtas AZ, Paschalis V, Fatouros IG, Koutedakis Y, Kouretas D. The effect of muscle-damaging exercise on blood and skeletal muscle oxidative stress: magnitude and time-course considerations. Sports Med. 2008;38(7):579-606.

Packer L, Oxidants, antioxidant nutrients and the athlete. J Sports Sci. 1997 Jun;15(3):353-63.

Panza VS, Wazlawik E, Ricardo Schütz G, Comin L, Hecht KC, da Silva EL. Consumption of green tea favorably affects oxidative stress markers in weight-trained men. Nutrition. 2008 May;24(5):433-42. Epub 2008 Mar 12.

Quadrilatero J, Hoffman-Goetz L: N-Acetyl-L-Cysteine inhibits exercise-induced lymphocyte apoptotic protein alterations. Med Sci Sports Exerc 2005, 37(1):53-56.

Reid MB, Stokic DS, Koch SM, et al.: N-Acetylcysteine inhibits muscle fatigue in humans. J Clin Invest 1994, 94:2468-2474.

Ristow M, Zarse K, Oberbach A, Klöting N, Birringer M, Kiehntopf M, Stumvoll M, Kahn CR, Blüher M. Antioxidants prevent health-promoting effects of physical exercise in humans. Proc Natl Acad Sci U S A. 2009 May 26;106(21):8665-70. Epub 2009 May 11.

Sen CK, Packer L: Thiol homeostasis and supplements in physical exercise. Am J Clin Nutr 2000, 72(suppl):653S-669S.

Sen CK. Antioxidants in exercise nutrition. Sports Med. 2001;31(13):891-908.

Sen CK: Glutathione homeostasis in response to exercise training and nutritional supplements. Molecular and Cellular Biochemistry 1999, 196:31-42.

Senturk UK, Yalcin O, Gunduz F, Kuru O, Meiselman HJ, Baskurt OK. Effect of antioxidant vitamin treatment on the time course of hematological and hemorheological alterations after an exhausting exercise episode in human subjects. J Appl Physiol. 2005 Apr;98(4):1272-9. Epub 2004 Dec 3.

Sharman JE, Endurance exercise, plasma oxidation and cardiovascular risk. Acta Cardiol. 2004 Dec;59(6):636-42

Supinski GS, Stofan D, Ciufo R, et al.: N-acetylcysteine administration alters the response to inspiratory loading in oxygensupplemented rats. J Appl Physiol 1997, 82(4):1119-1125

Tauler P, Ferrer MD, Sureda A, Pujol P, Drobnic F, Tur JA, Pons A. Supplementation with an antioxidant cocktail containing coenzyme Q prevents plasma oxidative damage induced by soccer. Eur J Appl Physiol. 2008 Nov;104(5):777-85. Epub 2008 Jul 30.

Tecklenburg SL, Mickleborough TD, Fly AD, Bai Y, Stager JM. Ascorbic acid supplementation attenuates exercise-induced bronchoconstriction in patients with asthma. Respir Med. 2007 Aug;101(8):1770-8. Epub 2007 Apr 5.

Vina J, Gomez-Cabrera MC, Lloret A, Marquez R, Minana JB, Pallardo FV, Sastre J. Free radicals in exhaustive physical exercise: mechanism of production, and protection by antioxidants. IUBMB Life. 2000 Oct-Nov;50(4-5):271-7.

Wang H, Nair MG, Strasburg GM, Chang YC, Booren AM, Gray JI, DeWitt

DL: Antioxidant and antiinflammatory activities of anthocyanins and their aglycon, cyanidin, from tart cherries. J Nat Prod 1999, 62:802.

Watson TA, Callister R, Taylor R, Sibbritt D, MacDonald-Wicks LK, Garg ML. Antioxidant restricted diet increases oxidative stress during acute exhaustive exercise. Asia Pac J Clin Nutr. 2003;12 Suppl:S9.

Zembron-Lacny A, Slowinska-Lisowska M, Szygula Z, Witkowski K, Szyszka K. The comparison of antioxidant and hematological properties of N-acetylcysteine and alpha-lipoic acid in physically active males. Physiol Res. 2009;58(6):855-61. Epub 2008 Dec 17.

Zembron-Lacny A, Slowinska-Lisowska M, Szygula Z, Witkowski K, Stefaniak T, Dziubek W. Assessment of the antioxidant effectiveness of alpha-lipoic acid in healthy men exposed to muscle-damaging exercise. J Physiol Pharmacol. 2009 Jun;60(2):139-43.

Zembron-Lacny A, Ostapiuk J, Szyszka K. Effects of sulphur-containing compounds on plasma redox status in muscle-damaging exercise. Chin J Physiol. 2009 Oct 31;52(5):289-94.

Zembron-Lacny A, Szyszka K, Szygula Z. Effect of cysteine derivatives administration in healthy men exposed to intense resistance exercise by evaluation of pro-antioxidant ratio. J Physiol Sci. 2007 Dec;57(6):343-8. Epub 2007 Nov 15.

Zoppi CC, Hohl R, Silva FC, Lazarim FL, Neto JM, Stancanneli M, Macedo DV.Vitamin C and e supplementation effects in professional soccer players under regular training. J Int Soc Sports Nutr. 2006 Dec 13;3:37-44.

Chapter 4

Arnaud, Alexandra, López-Pedrosa, José María, Torres, María Isabel, Gil, Ángel, Dietary Nucleotides Modulate Mitochondrial Function of Intestinal Mucosa in Weanling Rats with Chronic Diarrhea Journal of Pediatric Gastroenterology & Nutrition: August 2003 - Volume 37 - Issue 2 - pp 124-131

Artioli GG, Gualano B, Smith A, Stout J, Lancha AH Jr. Role of beta-alanine supplementation on muscle carnosine and exercise performance. Med Sci Sports Exerc. 2010 Jun;42(6):1162-73.

Baguet A, Koppo K, Pottier A, Derave W. Beta-alanine supplementation reduces acidosis but not oxygen uptake response during high-intensity cycling exercise. Eur J Appl Physiol. 2010 Feb;108(3):495-503.

Blomstrand E.J, A role for branched-chain amino acids in reducing central fatigue. Nutr. 2006 Feb;136(2):544S-547S.

Brault JJ, Towse TF, Slade JM, Meyer RA. Parallel increases in phosphocreatine and total creatine in human vastus lateralis muscle during creatine supplementation. Int J Sport Nutr Exerc Metab. 2007 Dec;17(6):624-34.

Brault JJ and Terjung RL. Purine salvage to adenine nucleotides in different skeletal muscle fiber types. *J Appl Physiol* 91: 231–238, 2001.

Burke DG, Chilibeck PD, Parise G, Tarnopolsky MA, Candow DG. Effect of alpha-lipoic acid combined with creatine monohydrate on human skeletal muscle creatine and phosphagen concentration. Int J Sport Nutr Exerc Metab. 2003 Sep;13(3):294-302.

Cooke M, Iosia M, Buford T, Shelmadine B, Hudson G, Kerksick C, Rasmussen C, Greenwood M, Leutholtz B, Willoughby D, Kreider R. Effects of acute and 14-day coenzyme Q10 supplementation on exercise performance in both trained and untrained individuals. J Int Soc Sports Nutr. 2008 Mar 4;5:8.

Coombes JS, Rowell B, Dodd SL, Demirel HA, Naito H, Shanely RA, Powers SK. Effects of vitamin E deficiency on fatigue and muscle contractile properties. Eur J Appl Physiol 2002; 87(3):272-277

Cruzat VF, Rogero MM, Tirapegui J. Effects of supplementation with free glutamine and the dipeptide Alanyl glutamine on parameters of muscle damage and inflammation in rats submitted to prolonged exercise. Cell Biochemistry & Function. 28(1):24-30, 2010

Davis JM, Carlstedt CJ, Chen S, Carmichael MD, Murphy EA. The dietary flavonoid quercetin increases VO(2max) and endurance capacity. Int J Sport Nutr Exerc Metab. 2010 Feb;20(1):56-62.

Davis JM, et al, Effects of Branched-Chain Amino Acids and Carbohydrate on Fatigue During Intermittent, High-Intensity Running, Int J Sports Med, 1999;20:309-314

Dechent, P., Pouwels, P. J. W., Wilken, B., Hanefeld, F. & Frahm, J. 1999 Increase of total creatine in human brain after oral supplementation of creatine-monohydrate. Am. J. Physiol. **277**, R698–R704.

Derave W, Everaert I, Beeckman S, Baguet A. Muscle carnosine metabolism and beta-alanine supplementation in relation to exercise and training. Sports Med. 2010 Mar 1;40(3):247-63.

Decorte N, Lafaix PA, Millet GY, Wuyam B, Verges S. Scand J Med Sci

Sports. 2010 Aug 30. Central and peripheral fatigue kinetics during exhaustive constant-load cycling.

Enoka RM, Stuart DG. Neurobiology of muscle fatigue. J Appl Physiol 1992; 72(5):1631-1638.

Fernström M, Bakkman L, Tonkonogi M, Shabalina IG, Rozhdestvenskaya Z, Mattsson CM, Enqvist JK, Ekblom B, Sahlin K. Reduced efficiency, but increased fat oxidation, in mitochondria from human skeletal muscle after 24-h ultraendurance exercise. J Appl Physiol. 2007 May;102(5):1844-9. Epub 2007 Jan 18.

Giannini Artioli G, Gualano B, Smith A, Stout J, Herbert Lancha A Junior. The Role of beta-alanine Supplementation on Muscle Carnosine and Exercise Performance. Med Sci Sports Exerc. 2009 Dec 9.

Graham TE. Caffeine and exercise: metabolism, endurance and performance. Sports Med 2001; 31(11):785-807

Gökbel H, Gül I, Belviranl M, Okudan N. The effects of coenzyme Q10 supplementation on performance during repeated bouts of supramaximal exercise in sedentary men. J Strength Cond Res. 2010 Jan;24(1):97-102.

Hellsten Y, Richter EA, Kiens B, and Bangsbo J. AMP deamination and purine exchange in human skeletal muscle during and after intense exercise. *J Physiol* 20: 909–920, 1999

Hellsten-Westing Y, Balsom PD, Norman B, and Sjödin B. The effect of high-intensity training on purine metabolism in man. *Acta Physiol Scand* 149: 405–412, 1993

Hellsten, L. Skadhauge, and J. Bangsbo Effect of ribose supplementation on resynthesis of adenine nucleotides after intense intermittent training in humans, *Am J Physiol Regul Integr Comp Physiol* 286: R182–R188, 2004;

Hellsten Y, Skadhauge L, Bangsbo J. Effect of ribose supplementation on resynthesis of adenine nucleotides after intense intermittent training in humans. Am J Physiol Regul Integr Comp Physiol. 2004 Jan;286(1):R182-8.

Ho JY, Kraemer WJ, Volek JS, Fragala MS, Thomas GA, Dunn-Lewis C, Coday M, Häkkinen K, Maresh CM. L-carnitine L-tartrate supplementation favorably affects biochemical markers of recovery from physical exertion in middle-aged men and women. Metabolism Clinical and Experimental (2010) –In Press

Hoffman J, Ratamess NA, Ross R, Kang J, Magrelli J, Neese K, Faigenbaum AD, Wise JA. Beta-alanine and the hormonal response to exercise. Int J Sports Med. 2008 Dec;29(12):952-8. Epub 2008 Jun 11.

Hoffman, J.R., et al., Examination of the efficacy of acute L-alanyl-L-glutamine ingestion during hydration stress in endurance exercise. J Int Soc Sports Nutr. 7: p. 8. 2010.

Jones AM, Wilkerson DP, Fulford J. Influence of dietary creatine supplementation on muscle phosphocreatine kinetics during knee-extensor exercise in humans. Am J Physiol Regul Integr Comp Physiol. 2009 Apr;296(4):R1078-87

Jordan T, Lukaszuk J, Misic M, Umoren J. Effect of beta-alanine supplementation on the onset of blood lactate accumulation (OBLA) during treadmill running: Pre/post 2 treatment experimental design. J Int Soc Sports Nutr. 2010 May 19;7:20.

Kendrick IP, Kim HJ, Harris RC, Kim CK, Dang VH, Lam TQ, Bui TT, Wise JA. The effect of 4 weeks beta-alanine supplementation and isokinetic training on carnosine concentrations in type I and II human skeletal muscle fibres. Eur J Appl Physiol. 2009 May;106(1):131-8. Epub 2009 Feb 12.

Koba T, Hamada K, et al., Branched-chain amino acids supplementation attenuates the accumulation of blood lactate dehydrogenase during distance running,", J Sports Med Phys Fitness, 2007; 47(3): 316-322

Kon M, Tanabe K, Akimoto T, Kimura F, Tanimura Y, Shimizu K, Okamoto T, Kono I. Reducing exercise-induced muscular injury in kendo athletes with supplementation of coenzyme Q10. Br J Nutr. 2008 Oct;100(4):903-9. Epub 2008 Feb 20.

Kraemer WJ, Spiering BA, Volek JS, Ratamess NA, Sharman MJ, Rubin MR, French DN, Silvestre R, Hatfield DL, Van Heest JL, Vingren JL, Judelson DA, Deschenes MR, Maresh CM Androgenic responses to resistance exercise: effects of feeding and L-carnitine. Med Sci Sports Exerc. 2006 Jul;38(7):1288-96.

Kraemer WJ, Volek JS, French DN, Rubin MR, Sharman MJ, Gómez AL, Ratamess NA, Newton RU, Jemiolo B, Craig BW, Häkkinen K. The effects of L-carnitine L-tartrate supplementation on hormonal responses to resistance exercise and recovery. J Strength Cond Res. 2003 Aug;17(3):455-62.

Lambert CP, Flynn MG. Fatigue during High-Intensity Intermittent Exercise: Application to Bodybuilding. Sports Med 2002; 32(8):511-522.

Lima AA. Carvalho GH. Figueiredo AA. Gifoni AR. Soares AM. Silva EA. Guerrant RL. Effects of an alanyl-glutamine-based oral rehydration and nutrition therapy solution on electrolyte and water absorption in a rat model of secretory diarrhea induced by cholera toxin. Nutrition. 18(6):458-62, 2002

Littarru GP, Tiano L. Clinical aspects of coenzyme Q10: an update. Nutrition. 2010 Mar;26(3):250-4. Epub 2009 Nov 22.

Lyadurai SJ, Chung SS.New-onset seizures in adults: possible association with consumption of popular energy drinks. Epilepsy Behav. 2007 May;10(3):504-8. Epub 2007 Mar 8.

MacDougall JD, Ray S, Sale DG McCartney N, Lee P, Garner S. Muscle substrate utilization and lactate production during weightlifting. Canadian Journal of Applied Physiology 1999; 24:209-215.

Martin V, Kerhervé H, Messonnier LA, Banfi JC, Geyssant A, Bonnefoy R, Féasson L, Millet GY., Central and peripheral contributions to neuromuscular fatigue induced by a 24-h treadmill run. J Appl Physiol. 2010 May;108(5):1224-33

Mizuno K, Tanaka M, Nozaki S, Mizuma H, Ataka S, Tahara T, Sugino T, Shirai T, Kajimoto Y, Kuratsune H, Kajimoto O, Watanabe Y. Antifatigue effects of coenzyme Q10 during physical fatigue. Nutrition. 2008 Apr;24(4):293-9. Epub 2008 Feb 13.

Newcomer BR, Exercise over-stress and maximal muscle oxidative metabolism using magnetic resonance spectroscopy Br J Sports Med. 2005 May;39(5):302-6

Pan JW, Takahashi K. Cerebral energetic effects of creatine supplementation in humans. Am J Physiol Regul Integr Comp Physiol. 2007 Apr;292(4):R1745-50

Pérez MJ, Sánchez-Medina F, Torres M, Gil A, Suárez A. Dietary nucleotides enhance the liver redox state and protein synthesis in cirrhotic rats. J Nutr. 2004 Oct;134(10):2504-8.

Rennie MJ, Bohé J, Smith K, Wackerhage H, Greenhaff P Branched-chain amino acids as fuels and anabolic signals in human muscle. J Nutr. 2006 Jan;136(1 Suppl):264S-8S.

Sale C, Saunders B, Harris RC. Effect of beta-alanine supplementation on muscle carnosine concentrations and exercise performance. Amino Acids. 2010 Jul;39(2):321-33. Epub 2009 Dec 20.

Schoch RD, Willoughby D, Greenwood M. The regulation and expression of the creatine transporter: a brief review of creatine supplementation in humans and animals. J Int Soc Sports Nutr. 2006 Jun 23;3:60-6.

Shimomura, Y. Murakami, T.Nakai, N. Nagasaki, M. Harri, R.A. (2004). Exercise Promotes BCAA Catabolism: Effects of BCAA Supplementation on Skeletal Muscle during Exercise J. Nutri. 134: 1583S-1587S

Skurvydas A, Brazaitis M, Kamandulis S, Sipaviciene, S, Peripheral and central fatigue after muscle-damaging exercise is muscle length dependent and inversely related. J Electromyogr Kinesiol. 2010 Aug;20(4):655-60

Skurvydas A, Brazaitis M, Streckis V, Rudas E. The effect of plyometric training on central and peripheral fatigue in boys. Int J Sports Med. 2010 Jul;31(7):451-7.

Smith AE, Walter AA, Graef JL, Kendall KL, Moon JR, Lockwood CM, Fukuda DH, Beck TW, Cramer JT, Stout JR. Effects of beta-alanine supplementation and high-intensity interval training on endurance performance and body composition in men; a double-blind trial. J Int Soc Sports Nutr. 2009 Feb 11;6:5.

Spiering BA, Kraemer WJ, Hatfield DL, Vingren JL, Fragala MS, Ho JY, Thomas GA, Häkkinen K, Volek JS. Effects of L-carnitine L-tartrate supplementation on muscle oxygenation responses to resistance exercise. J Strength Cond Res. 2008 Jul;22(4):1130-5.

Spiering BA, Kraemer WJ, Vingren JL, Hatfield DL, Fragala MS, Ho JY, Maresh CM, Anderson JM, Volek JS. Responses of criterion variables to different supplemental doses of L-carnitine L-tartrate. J Strength Cond Res. 2007 Feb;21(1):259-64.

St Clair Gibson A, Lambert MI, Weston AR, Myburgh KH, Emms M, Kirby P, Marinaki AM, Owen PE, Derman W, Noakes TD. Exercise-induced mitochondrial dysfunction in an elite athlete. Clin J Sport Med. 1998 Jan;8(1):52-5.

Sugita M, Ohtani M, Ishii N, Maruyama K, Kobayashi K. Effect of a selected amino acid mixture on the recovery from muscle fatigue during and after eccentric contraction exercise training. Biosci Biotechnol Biochem. 2003 Feb;67(2):372-5.

Tauler P, Ferrer MD, Sureda A, Pujol P, Drobnic F, Tur JA, Pons A. Supplementation with an antioxidant cocktail containing coenzyme Q prevents plasma oxidative damage induced by soccer. Eur J Appl Physiol. 2008 Nov;104(5):777-85. Epub 2008 Jul 30.

Teitelbaum JE, Johnson C., The use of D-ribose in chronic fatigue syndrome and fibromyalgia: a pilot study. J Altern Complement Med. 2006 Nov;12(9):857-62.

Triscott S, Gordon J, Kuppuswamy A, King N, Davey N, Ellaway P. J Sports Sci. 2008 Jul;26(9):941-51. Differential effects of endurance and resistance training on central fatigue.

Van Thienen R, Van Proeyen K, Vanden Eynde B, Puype J, Lefere T, Hespel P. Beta-alanine improves sprint performance in endurance cycling. Med Sci Sports Exerc. 2009 Apr;41(4):898-903.

Vandenberghe K, Goris M, Van Hecke P, Van Leemputte M, Vangerven L, Hespel P. Long-term creatine intake is beneficial to muscle performance during resistance training. Journal of Applied Physiology 1997; 83:2055-2063.

Volek JS, Kraemer WJ, Rubin MR, Gómez AL, Ratamess NA, Gaynor P. L-Carnitine L-tartrate supplementation favorably affects markers of recovery from exercise stress. Am J Physiol Endocrinol Metab. 2002 Feb;282(2):E474-82.

Volek JS, Kraemer WJ, Bush JA et al. Creatine supplementation enhances muscular performance during high-intensity resistance exercise. Journal of the American Dietetic Association 1997;97:765-770.

Watanabe A, Kato N, Kato T. Effects of creatine on mental fatigue and cerebral hemoglobin oxygenation. Neurosci Res 2002 Apr;42(4):279-85.

Weir JP, Beck TW, Cramer JT, Housh TJ. Is fatigue all in your head? A critical review of the central governor model. Br J Sports Med. 2006 Jul;40(7):573-86; discussion 586.

Zarzeczny R, Brault JJ, Abraham KA, Hancock CR, and Terjung R. Influence of ribose on adenine salvage after intense muscle contractions. *J Appl Physiol* 91: 1775–1781, 2001

Zheng A, Moritani T. Influence of CoQ10 on autonomic nervous activity and energy metabolism during exercise in healthy subjects. J Nutr Sci Vitaminol (Tokyo). 2008 Aug;54(4):286-90.

Chapter 5

Apró W, Blomstrand E. Influence of supplementation with branched-chain amino acids in combination with resistance exercise on p70S6 kinase phosphorylation in resting and exercising human skeletal muscle. Acta Physiol (Oxf). 2010 Nov;200(3):237-48.

Atassi N, Ratai EM, Greenblatt DJ, Pulley D, Zhao Y, Bombardier J, Wallace S, Eckenrode J, Cudkowicz M, Dibernardo A. A phase I, pharmacokinetic, dosage escalation study of creatine monohydrate in subjects with amyotrophic lateral sclerosis. Amyotroph Lateral Scler. 2010 Aug 11.

Baier S, Johannsen D, Abumrad N, Rathmacher JA, Nissen S, Flakoll P. Year-long changes in protein metabolism in elderly men and women supplemented with a nutrition cocktail of beta-hydroxy-beta-methylbutyrate (HMB), L-arginine, and L-lysine. JPEN J Parenter Enteral Nutr. 2009 Jan-Feb;33(1):71-82.

Bailey SJ, Winyard PG, Vanhatalo A, Blackwell JR, DiMenna FJ, Wilkerson DP, Jones AM. Acute L-arginine supplementation reduces the O2 cost of moderate-intensity exercise and enhances high-intensity exercise tolerance. J Appl Physiol. 2010 Nov;109(5):1394-403. Epub 2010 Aug 19.

Barnes MJ, Mündel T, Stannard SR. Acute alcohol consumption aggravates the decline in muscle performance following strenuous eccentric exercise. J Sci Med Sport. 2010 Jan;13(1):189-93.

Bassini-Cameron A, Monteiro A, Gomes A, Werneck-de-Castro JP, Cameron L. Glutamine protects against increases in blood ammonia in football players in an exercise intensity-dependent way. Br J Sports Med. 2008 Apr;42(4):260-6. Epub 2007 Nov 5.

Béard E, Braissant O. Synthesis and transport of creatine in the CNS: importance for cerebral functions. J Neurochem. 2010 Jul 29.

Blonde-Cynober, Use of ornithine -ketoglutarate in clinical nutrition of elderly patients., Nutrition, Volume 19, Issue 1 p73-75, January 2003

Blomstrand E, Eliasson J, Karlsson HK, Köhnke R. Branched-chain amino acids activate key enzymes in protein synthesis after physical exercise. J Nutr. 2006 Jan;136(1 Suppl):269S-73S.

Borsheim E, Aarsland A, Wolfe RR. Effect of an amino acid, protein, and carbohydrate mixture on net muscle protein balance after resistance exercise. Int J Sport Nutr Exerc Metab. 2004 Jun;14(3):255-71.

Børsheim E, Cree MG, Tipton KD, Elliott TA, Aarsland A, Wolfe RR. Effect of carbohydrate intake on net muscle protein synthesis during recovery from resistance exercise. J Appl Physiol. 2004 Feb;96(2):674-8. Epub 2003 Oct 31.

Brosnan JT, Brosnan ME. Creatine metabolism and the urea cycle. Mol Genet Metab. 2010;100 Suppl 1:S49-52. Epub 2010 Mar 1.

Buckley JD, Thomson RL, Coates AM, Howe PR, DeNichilo MO, Rowney MK Supplementation with a whey protein hydrolysate enhances recovery of muscle force-generating capacity following eccentric exercise. J Sci Med Sport. 2010 Jan;13(1):178-81.

Buchman AL. Glutamine: commercially essential or conditionally essential? A critical appraisal of the human data. Am J Clin Nutr. 2001;74(1):25-32.

Camic CL, Housh TJ, Mielke M, Zuniga JM, Hendrix CR, Johnson GO, Schmidt RJ, Housh DJ. The effects of 4 weeks of an arginine-based supplement on the gas exchange threshold and peak oxygen uptake. Appl Physiol Nutr Metab. 2010 Jun;35(3):286-93.

Camic CL, Housh TJ, Zuniga JM, Hendrix RC, Mielke M, Johnson GO, Schmidt RJ Effects of arginine-based supplements on the physical working capacity at the fatigue threshold. J Strength Cond Res. 2010 May;24(5):1306-12.

Castell LM, Newsholme EA. The effects of oral glutamine supplementation on athletes after prolonged, exhaustive exercise. Nutrition 1997;13:738-42.

Chen S, Kim W, Henning SM, Carpenter CL, Li Z. Arginine and antioxidant supplement on performance in elderly male cyclists: a randomized controlled trial. J Int Soc Sports Nutr. 2010 Mar 23;7:13. Clarkson, P.M., & Hubal, M.J., Exercise-induced muscle damage in humans. American Journal of Physical Medicine and Rehabilitation 2002 (81) (Suppl), S52-S69.

Clarkson, PM, Tremblay, I., Exercise-induced muscle damage and rapid adaptation in humans. Journal of Applied Physiology 1998, 65(1) 1-6.

Collier SR, Collins E, Kanaley JA. Oral arginine attenuates the growth hormone response to resistance exercise. J Appl Physiol. 2006 Sep;101(3):848-52. Epub 2006 Jun 1.

Cooke MB, Rybalka E, Stathis CG, Cribb PJ, Hayes A. Whey protein isolate attenuates strength decline after eccentrically-induced muscle damage in healthy individuals. J Int Soc Sports Nutr. 2010 Sep 22;7:30.

Coudray-Lucas C, Le Bever H, Cynober L, De Bandt JP, Carsin H. Ornithine alpha-ketoglutarate improves wound healing in severe burn patients:

a prospective randomized double-blind trial versus isonitrogenous controls. Crit Care Med. 2000 Jun;28(6):1772-6.

Cynober L, Moinard C, De Bandt JP. The 2009 ESPEN Sir David Cuthbertson. Citrulline: a new major signaling molecule or just another player in the pharmaconutrition game? Clin Nutr. 2010 Oct;29(5):545-51. Epub 2010 Aug 16.

Cynober L, Lasnier E, Le Boucher J, Jardel A, Coudray-Lucas C. Effect of ornithine alpha-ketoglutarate on glutamine pools in burn injury: evidence of component interaction. Intensive Care Med. 2007 Mar;33(3):538-41. Epub 2007 Jan 18.

Cynober L. Ornithine alpha-ketoglutarate as a potent precursor of arginine and nitric oxide: a new job for an old friend. J Nutr. 2004 Oct;134(10 Suppl):2858S-2862S; discussion 2895S.

Cynober LA., The use of alpha-ketoglutarate salts in clinical nutrition and metabolic care., Curr Opin Clin Nutr Metab Care. 1999 Jan;2(1):33-7.

De Bandt JP, Coudray-Lucas C, Lioret N, Lim SK, Saizy R, Giboudeau J, Cynober L., A randomized controlled trial of the influence of the mode of enteral ornithine alpha-ketoglutarate administration in burn patients., J Nutr. 1998 Mar;128(3):563-9.

Demarcq JM, Delbar M, Trochu G, Crignon JJ., Effects of ornithine alpha-ketoglutarate on the nutritional state of intensive-care patients., Cah Anesthesiol. 1984 Mar;32(3):229-32.

Ding C, Cicuttini F, Jones G. Do NSAIDs affect longitudinal changes in knee cartilage volume and knee cartilage defects in older adults? Am J Med. 2009 Sep;122(9):836-42.

Donati L, Ziegler F, Pongelli G, Signorini MS., Nutritional and clinical efficacy of ornithine alpha-ketoglutarate in severe burn patients., Clin Nutr. 1999 Oct;18(5):307-11

Erin L. Glynn, Christopher S. Fry, Micah J. Drummond, Hans C. Dreyer, Shaheen Dhanani, Elena Volpi, and Blake B. Rasmussen, Muscle Protein Breakdown has a Minor Role in the Protein Anabolic Response to Essential Amino Acid and Carbohydrate Intake Following Resistance Exercise Am J Physiol Regul Integr Comp Physiol (June 2, 2010)

Frassetto, L. et al. Estimation of net endongenous noncarbonic acid production in humans from diet potassium and protein contents. Am J Clin Nutr, 1998;68:576-83.

Gleeson M. Dosing and efficacy of glutamine supplementation in human exercise and sport training. J Nutr. 2008 Oct;138(10):2045S-2049S.

Gualano B, Ferreira DC, Sapienza MT, Seguro AC, Lancha AH Jr. Effect of short-term high-dose creatine supplementation on measured GFR in a young man with a single kidney. Am J Kidney Dis. 2010 Mar;55(3):e7-9. Epub 2010 Jan 8.

Gualano B, de Salles Painelli V, Roschel H, Lugaresi R, Dorea E, Artioli GG, Lima FR, da Silva ME, Cunha MR, Seguro AC, Shimizu MH, Otaduy MC, Sapienza MT, da Costa Leite C, Bonfá E, Lancha Junior AH. Creatine supplementation does not impair kidney function in type 2 diabetic patients: a randomized, double-blind, placebo-controlled, clinical trial. Eur J Appl Physiol. 2010 Oct 26.

Fukuda DH, Smith AE, Kendall KL, Dwyer TR, Kerksick CM, Beck TW, Cramer JT, Stout JR. The effects of creatine loading and gender on anaerobic running capacity. J Strength Cond Res. 2010 Jul;24(7):1826-33.

Gualano B, de Salles Painneli V, Roschel H, Artioli GG, Junior MN, Lúcia de Sá Pinto A, Rossi da Silva ME, Cunha MR, Otaduy MC, da Costa Leite C, Ferreira JC, Pereira RM, Brum PC, Bonfá E, Lancha AH Junior. Creatine in Type 2 Diabetes: A Randomized, Double-Blind, Placebo-Controlled Trial. Med Sci Sports Exerc. 2010 Sep 24.

Haraguchi FK, et al., Evaluation of Biological and Biochemical Quality of Whey Protein. J Med Food. 2010 Sep 27

Hammarqvist F, Wernerman J, Ali R, Vinnars E., Effects of an amino acid solution enriched with either branched chain amino acids or ornithine-alpha-ketoglutarate on the postoperative intracellular amino acid concentration of skeletal muscle., Br J Surg. 1990 Feb;77(2):214-8.

Howatson G, van Someren KA. The prevention and treatment of exercise-induced muscle damage. Sports Med. 2008;38(6):483-503.

Hulmi JJ, Lockwood CM, Stout JR., Effect of protein/essential amino acids and resistance training on skeletal muscle hypertrophy: A case for whey protein. Nutr Metab (Lond). 2010 Jun 17;7:51.

Ivy JL, Early postexercise muscle glycogen recovery is enhanced with a carbohydrate-protein supplement. Carb:Protein Ratio (4:1, 3:1) J Appl Physiol. 2002 Oct;93(4):1337-44.

Iwashita S, Williams P, Jabbour K, Ueda T, Kobayashi H, Baier S, Flakoll PJ. Impact of glutamine supplementation on glucose homeostasis during and after exercise. J Appl Physiol. 2005 Nov;99(5):1858-65. Epub 2005 Jul 21.

Jeevanandam M, Petersen SR., Substrate fuel kinetics in enterally fed trauma patients supplemented with ornithine alpha ketoglutarate., Clin Nutr. 1999 Aug;18(4):209-17.

Kanaley JA. Growth hormone, arginine and exercise. Curr Opin Clin Nutr Metab Care. 2008 Jan;11(1):50-4.

Kargotich S, Goodman C, Dawson B, Morton AR, Keast D, Joske DJ. Plasma glutamine responses to high-intensity exercise before and after endurance training. Res Sports Med. 2005 Oct-Dec;13(4):287-300.

Kraemer WJ, Volek JS, French DN, Rubin MR, Sharman MJ, Gómez AL, Ratamess NA, Newton RU, Jemiolo B, Craig BW, Häkkinen K. The effects of L-carnitine L-tartrate supplementation on hormonal responses to resistance exercise and recovery. J Strength Cond Res. 2003 Aug;17(3):455-62.

Krista R Howarth, Regulation of human skeletal muscle protein metabolism: Effect of exercise, nutrition and physical training, ETD Collection for McMaster University January 2007 Paper AAINR36046

Kuhls DA, Rathmacher JA, Musngi MD, Frisch DA, Nielson J, Barber A, MacIntyre AD, Coates JE, Fildes JJ. Beta-hydroxy-beta-methylbutyrate supplementation in critically ill trauma patients. J Trauma. 2007 Jan;62(1):125-31; discussion 131-2.

Lamboley CR, Royer D, Dionne IJ Effects of beta-hydroxy-beta-methylbutyrate on aerobic-performance components and body composition in college students. Int J Sport Nutr Exerc Metab. 2007 Feb;17(1):56-69.

Lane AR, Duke JW, Hackney AC. Influence of dietary carbohydrate intake on the free testosterone: cortisol ratio responses to short-term intensive exercise training. Eur J Appl Physiol. 2010 Apr;108(6):1125-31. Epub 2009 Dec 20.

Lemann J Jr. Relationship between urinary calcium and net acid excretion as determined by dietary protein and potassium: a review. Nephron 1999;81(suppl):18 –25

Liu TH, Wu CL, Chiang CW, Lo YW, Tseng HF, Chang CK. No effect of short-term arginine supplementation on nitric oxide production, metabolism and performance in intermittent exercise in athletes. J Nutr Biochem. 2009 Jun;20(6):462-8. Epub 2008 Aug 15.

J Gerontol A Biol Sci Med Sci. 1999 Aug;54(8):M395-9. Oral arginine does not stimulate basal or augment exercise-induced GH secretion in either young or old adults. Marcell TJ, Taaffe DR, Hawkins SA, Tarpenning KM, Pyka G, Kohlmeier L, Wiswell RA, Marcus R.

Matsumoto K, Mizuno M, Mizuno T, Dilling-Hansen B, Lahoz A, Bertelsen V, Münster H, Jordening H, Hamada K, Doi T. Branched-chain amino acids and arginine supplementation attenuates skeletal muscle proteolysis induced by moderate exercise in young individuals. Int J Sports Med. 2007 Jun;28(6):531-8. Epub 2007 May 11.

May PE, et al. Reversal of cancer-related wasting using oral supplementation with a combination of beta-hydroxy-beta-methylbutyrate, arginine, and glutamine. Am J Surg 2002;183:471-9.

Melis GC, ter Wengel N, Boelens PG, van Leeuwen PA. Glutamine: recent developments in research on the clinical significance of glutamine. Curr Opin Clin Nutr Metab Care. 2004 Jan;7(1):59-70. Review.

Miller AL. Therapeutic considerations of L-glutamine: a review of the literature. Altern Med Rev 1999;4:239-48.

Moore DR, Robinson MJ, Fry JL, Tang JE, Glover EI, Wilkinson SB, Prior T, Tarnopolsky MA, Phillips SM. Ingested protein dose response of muscle and albumin protein synthesis after resistance exercise in young men. Am J Clin Nutr. 2008 Dec 3.

Neu J, DeMarco V, Li N. Glutamine: clinical applications and mechanism of action. Curr Opin Clin Nutr Metab Care. 2002;5(1):69-75

Nunan D, Howatson G, van Someren KA. Exercise-induced muscle damage is not attenuated by beta-hydroxy-beta-methylbutyrate and alpha-ketoisocaproic acid supplementation. J Strength Cond Res. 2010 Feb;24(2):531-7.

O'Connor DM, Crowe MJ Effects of six weeks of beta-hydroxy-beta-methylbutyrate (HMB) and HMB/creatine supplementation on strength, power, and anthropometry of highly trained athletes. J Strength Cond Res. 2007 May;21(2):419-23.

Okutsu M, Suzuki K, Ishijima T, Peake J, Higuchi M. The effects of acute exercise-induced cortisol on CCR2 expression on human monocytes. Brain Behav Immun. 2008 Oct;22(7):1066-71. Epub 2008 May 13.

Pérez-Guisado J, Jakeman PM. Citrulline malate enhances athletic anaerobic performance and relieves muscle soreness. J Strength Cond Res. 2010 May;24(5):1215-22.

Portal S, Eliakim A, Nemet D, Halevy O, Zadik Z. Effect of HMB supplementation on body composition, fitness, hormonal profile and muscle damage indices. J Pediatr Endocrinol Metab. 2010 Jul;23(7):641-50.

Rahman ZA, Abdullah N, Singh R, Sosroseno W. Effect of acute exercise on the levels of salivary cortisol, tumor necrosis factor-alpha and nitric oxide. J Oral Sci. 2010;52(1):133-6.

Rathmacher JA, Nissen S, Panton L, Clark RH, Eubanks May P, Barber AE, D'Olimpio J, Abumrad NN. Supplementation with a combination of beta-hydroxy-beta-methylbutyrate (HMB), arginine, and glutamine is safe and could improve hematological parameters. JPEN J Parenter Enteral Nutr. 2004 Mar-Apr;28(2):65-75.

Rawson ES, Stec MJ, Frederickson SJ, Miles MP. Low-dose creatine supplementation enhances fatigue resistance in the absence of weight gain. Nutrition. 2010 Jun 29.

Rowlands DS, Thomson JS. Effects of beta-hydroxy-beta-methylbutyrate supplementation during resistance training on strength, body composition, and muscle damage in trained and untrained young men: a meta-analysis. J Strength Cond Res. 2009 May;23(3):836-46.

Sale C, Saunders B, Harris RC. Effect of beta-alanine supplementation on muscle carnosine concentrations and exercise performance. Amino Acids. 2010 Jul;39(2):321-33. Epub 2009 Dec 20.

Sarah B Wilkinson, Impact of resistance and endurance exercise and ingestion of varying protein sources on changes in human skeletal muscle protein turnover, ETD Collection for McMaster University January 2008, Paper AAINR57290

Stevenson, E., Williams, C. & Biscoe, H., The metabolic responses to high carbohydrate meals with different glycemic indices consumed during recovery from prolonged strenuous exercise. International Journal of Sport Nutrition and Exercise Metabolism, (2005) 15, 291-307.

Sureda A, Córdova A, Ferrer MD, Pérez G, Tur JA, Pons A. L-citrulline-malate influence over branched chain amino acid utilization during exercise. Eur J Appl Physiol. 2010 Sep;110(2):341-51. Epub 2010 May 25

Tang JE, Lysecki PJ, Manolakos JJ, Macdonald MJ, Tarnopolsky MA, Phillips SMBolus Arginine Supplementation Affects neither Muscle Blood Flow nor Muscle Protein Synthesis in Young Men at Rest or After Resistance Exercise. J Nutr. 2010 Dec 29.

Tang JE, et al , Ingestion of whey hydrolysate, casein, or soy protein isolate: effects on mixed muscle protein synthesis at rest and following resistance exercise in young men.

J Appl Physiol. 2009 Sep;107(3):987-92

Tee, Jason C, Bosch, Andrew N, Lambert, Mike I. Metabolic Consequences of Exercise-Induced Muscle Damage **Sports Medicine** 2007, Volume 37, Number 10, pp. 827-836(10)

Thomas NE, Leyshon A, Hughes MG, Davies B, Graham M, Baker JS. The effect of anaerobic exercise on salivary cortisol, testosterone and immunoglobulin (A) in boys aged 15-16 years. Eur J Appl Physiol. 2009 Nov;107(4):455-61. Epub 2009 Aug 11.

Thomson JS, Watson PE, Rowlands DS. Effects of nine weeks of beta-hydroxy-beta- methylbutyrate supplementation on strength and body composition in resistance trained men. J Strength Cond Res. 2009 May;23(3):827-35.

Tsai PH, Tang TK, Juang CL, Chen KW, Chi CA, Hsu MC. Effects of arginine supplementation on post-exercise metabolic responses. Chin J Physiol. 2009 Jun 30;52(3):136-42.

Van Loon, Saris WH, Kruijshoop M, Wagenmakers AJ., Maximizing postexercise muscle glycogen synthesis: carbohydrate supplementation and the application of amino acid or protein hydrosylate mixtures. Am J Clin Nutr 2000; 72: 106-111

van Someren KA, Edwards AJ, Howatson G. Supplementation with beta-hydroxy-beta-methylbutyrate (HMB) and alpha-ketoisocaproic acid (KIC) reduces signs and symptoms of exercise-induced muscle damage in man. Int J Sport Nutr Exerc Metab. 2005 Aug;15(4):413-24.

Viru M, Hackney AC, Janson T, Karelson K, Viru A. Characterization of the cortisol response to incremental exercise in physically active young men. Acta Physiol Hung. 2008 Jun;95(2):219-27.

Walrand S. Ornithine alpha-ketoglutarate: could it be a new therapeutic option for sarcopenia? J Nutr Health Aging. 2010;14(7):570-7.

Warren GL, Ingalls CP, Lowe DA, Armstrong RB. What mechanisms contribute to the strength loss that occurs during and in the recovery from skeletal muscle injury? J Orthop Sports Phys Ther. 2002 Feb;32(2):58-64.

Wernerman J, Hammarqvist F, von der Decken A, Vinnars E., Ornithine-alpha-ketoglutarate improves skeletal muscle protein synthesis as assessed by ribosome analysis and nitrogen use after surgery. Ann Surg. 1987 Nov;206(5):674-8.

Wernerman J, Hammarkvist F, Ali MR, Vinnars E., Glutamine and ornithine-alpha-ketoglutarate but not branched-chain amino acids reduce the loss of muscle glutamine after surgical trauma., Metabolism. 1989 Aug;38(8 Suppl 1):63-6.

Wilson JM, Kim JS, Lee SR, Rathmacher JA, Dalmau B, Kingsley JD, Koch H, Manninen AH, Saadat R, Panton LB. Acute and timing effects of beta-hydroxy-beta-methylbutyrate (HMB) on indirect markers of skeletal muscle damage. Nutr Metab (Lond). 2009 Feb 4;6:6.

Wilson GJ, Wilson JM, Manninen AH. Effects of beta-hydroxy-beta-methylbutyrate (HMB) on exercise performance and body composition across varying levels of age, sex, and training experience: A review. Nutr Metab (Lond). 2008 Jan 3;5:1.

Zanchi NE, Gerlinger-Romero F, Guimarães-Ferreira L, de Siqueira Filho MA, Felitti V, Lira FS, Seelaender M, Lancha AH Jr. HMB supplementation: clinical and athletic performance-related effects and mechanisms of action. Amino Acids. 2010 Jul 6. [Epub ahead of print]

Zajac A, Poprzecki S, Zebrowska A, Chalimoniuk M, Langfort J. Arginine and ornithine supplementation increases growth hormone and insulin-like growth factor-1 serum levels after heavy-resistance exercise in strength-trained athletes. J Strength Cond Res. 2010 Apr;24(4):1082-90.

Zawadzki YM, Yaspelkis BB, Ivy JL., Carbohydrate-protein complex increases the rate of muscle glycogen storage after exercise. J Appl Physiol 1992; 72 (5): 1854-1859

Chapter 6

Aloia JF and Li-Ng M. Re: epidemic influenza and vitamin D. Epidemiol Infect. 2007. 135:1095-6.

Bloomer RJ, Larson DE, Fisher-Wellman KH, Galpin AJ, Schilling BK.

Effect of eicosapentaenoic and docosahexaenoic acid on resting and exercise-induced inflammatory and oxidative stress biomarkers: a randomized, placebo controlled, cross-over study Lipids Health Dis. 2009 Aug 19;8:36.

Bucci L, Unlu L: Proteins and amino acid supplements in exercise and sport. In *Energy-Yielding Macronutrients and Energy Metabolism in Sports Nutrition*. Boca Raton, FL: CRC Press; 2000:191-212.

Burke LM: Nutritional needs for exercise in the heat. Comp Biochem Physiol A Mol Integr Physiol 2001. 128(4):735-48.

Burke LM: Nutrition for post-exercise recovery. Aust J Sci Med Sport 1997. 29(1):3-10.

Campbell B, Kreider RB, Ziegenfuss T, La Bounty P, Roberts M, Burke D, Landis J, Lopez H, Antonio J: International Society of Sports Nutrition position stand: protein and exercise. J Int Soc Sports. 2007. 4:8.

Carli G, Bonifazi M, Lodi L, Lupo C, Martelli G, Viti A: Changes in the exercise-induced hormone response to branched chain amino acid administration. Eur J Appl Physiol Occup Physiol 1992. 64(3):272-7.

Clark M, Reed DB, Crouse SF, Armstrong RB. Pre- and post-season dietary intake, body composition, and performance indices of NCAA division I female soccer players. Int J Sport Nutr Exerc Metab. 2003 Sep;13(3):303-19.

Cox AJ, Gleeson M, Pyne DB, Callister R, Hopkins WG, and Fricker PA. Clinical and laboratory evaluation of upper respiratory symptoms in elite athletes. Clin J Sport Med. 2008. 18(5): 438-45.

David S Weigle, Patricia A Breen, Colleen C Matthys, Holly S Callahan, Kaatje E Meeuws, Verna R Burden and Jonathan Q Purnell. A high-protein diet induces sustained reductions in appetite, ad libitum caloric intake, and body weight despite compensatory changes in diurnal plasma leptin and ghrelin concentrations. American Journal of Clinical Nutrition, 2005;82(1), 41-48.

Davis JM, Carlstedt CJ, Chen S, Carmichael MD, Murphy EA.The Dietary Flavonoid Quercetin Increases VO2max and Endurance Capacity. Int J Sport Nutr Exerc Metab. 2010 Feb;20(1):56-62.

Elitzak, H. "Food Marketing Costs At A Glance." Food Marketing 2001; 24(3):47-48. Accessed at http://www.ers.usda.gov/publications/FoodReview/septdec01/FRv24i3g.pdf on October 25, 2010.

Hawley, J.A. and Burke, L.M. Peak Performance: Training and Nutritional Strategies for Sport. 1998. Sydney: Allen and Unwin.

Heaney S, O'Connor H, Gifford J, Naughton G. Comparison of strategies for assessing nutritional adequacy in elite female athletes' dietary intake. Int J Sport Nutr Exerc Metab. 2010 Jun;20(3):245-56.

Hinton PS, Sanford TC, Davidson MM, Yakushko OF, Beck NC. Nutrient intakes and dietary behaviors of male and female collegiate athletes Int J Sport Nutr Exerc Metab. 2004 Aug;14(4):389-405.

http://www.heart.org/HEARTORG/GettingHealthy/NutritionCenter/ Knowing-Your-Fats_UCM_305976_Article.jsp. Accessed on November 1, 2010.

http://www.ars.usda.gov/SP2UserFiles/Place/12355000/pdf/0506/usual_ nutrient_intake_vitD_ca_phos_mg_2005-06.pdf. Accessed on October 29, 2010.

Hu FB, Manson JE, Willett WC: Types of dietary fat and risk of coronary heart disease: a critical review. J Am Coll Nutr. 2001 Feb;20(1):5-19.

Iwao S, et al. Effects of meal frequency on body composition during weight control in boxers. Scand J Med Sci Sports. 1996 Oct;6(5):265-72.

Jackie L. Buell et al. Presence of Metabolic Syndrome in Football Linemen. Journal of Athletic Training 2008;43(6):608–616.

Jequier E: Pathways to obesity. Int J Obes Relat metab Disord 2002, 26 Suppl 2:S12-7.

Jeukendrup AE, et al. Oxidation of carbohydrate feedings during prolonged exercise: current thoughts, guidelines and directions for future research. Sports Med 2000;29:407-424.

Jonnalagadda SS, Rosenbloom CA, Skinner R. Dietary practices, attitudes, and physiological status of collegiate freshman football players. J Strength Cond Res. 2001 Nov;15(4):507-13

Kerksick C, Harvey T, Stout J, Campbell B, Wilborn C, Kreider R, Kalman D, Ziegenfuss T, Lopez H, landis J, Ivy J, Antonio J. International Society of Sports Nutrition position stand: Nutrient Timing. Journal of the International Society of Sports Nutrition. 2008.

Kraemer W J, Volek JS, Clark KL, et al: Influence of exercise training on physiological and performance changes with weight loss in men. Med Sci Sports Exerc 1999;31:1320-1329.

Kreider RB: Dietary supplements and the promotion of muscle growth with resistance exercise. Sports Med 1999. 27(2):97-110

Kreider R et al. ISSN position. ISSN exercise & sport nutrition review: research & recommendations. Journal of the International Society of Sports Nutrition *2010, 7*:7

Leachman Slawson D, McClanahan BS, Clemens LH, Ward KD, Klesges RC, Vukadinovich CM, Cantler ED. Food sources of calcium in a sample of African-American an Euro-American collegiate athletes. Int J Sport Nutr Exerc Metab. 2001 Jun;11(2):199-208.

Leutholtz B, Kreider R: Exercise and Sport Nutrition. *In Nutritional Health.* Totowa, NJ: Humana Press; 2001:207-39.

MacRae and Mefferd. Dietary Antioxidant Supplementation Combined with Quercetin Improves Cycling Time Trial Performance. Int J Sport Nutr Exerc Metab. 2006, 16, 405-419.

Maughan R. The athlete's diet: nutritional goals and dietary strategies. Proc Nutr Soc. 2002 Feb;61(1):87-96.

Meksawan K, Venkatraman JT, Awad AB, Pendergast DR. Effect of dietary fat intake and exercise on inflammatory mediators of the immune system in sedentary men and women J Am Coll Nutr. 2004 Aug;23(4):331-40.

Mickleborough TD, Lindley MR, Montgomery GS. Effect of fish oil-derived omega-3 polyunsaturated Fatty Acid supplementation on exercise-induced bronchoconstriction and immune function in athletes.Phys Sportsmed. 2008 Dec;36(1):11-7.

Nieman, D.C. Nutrition, exercise, and immune system function. Clinics in Sports Med. 1999. 18: 537-548.

Nieman DC: Influence of carbohydrate on the immune response to intensive, prolonged exercise. Exerc Immunol Rev 1998. 4:64-76.

Noakes M, Keogh JB, Foster PR, Clifton PM. Effect of an energy-restricted, high protein, low-fat diet relative to a conventional high-carbohydrate, low fat diet on weight loss, body composition, nutritional status, and biomarkers of cardiovascular health in obese women. American Journal of Clinical Nutrition. 2005; 81(6):1298-1306.

Quercetin Reduces Illness but Not Immune Perturbations After Intensive ExerciseMed Sci Sports Exerc., 2007 Sep; 39(9): 1561-9. Neiman, David, Henson, DA, et al. Appalachian State University Study, Boone, NC.

Seebohar B. Nutrition Periodization for Endurance Athletes. 2004. Bull Publishing Co

Burke L and Coyle E. Nutrition for Athletes. Journal of Sports Sciences. 2004. 22(1):39-55.

Simopoulos AP. Omega 3 Fatty Acids and Athletics. Current Sports Medicine Reports. 2007. 6:230-236.

Tartibian, B.H. Maleki, A. Abbasi"The effects of omega-3 supplementation on pulmonary function of young wrestlers during intensive training" Journal of Science and Medicine in Sport March 2010, Volume 13, Issue 2, Pages 281-286.

Tipton KD, Borsheim E, Wolf SE, Sanford AP, Wolfe RR: Acute response of net muscle protein balance reflects 24-h balance after exercise and amino acid ingestion. Am J Physiol Endocrinol Metab 2003. 284(1):E76-89

USDA. "What we eat in America". Report of the DGAC on the Dietary Guidelines for Americans, 2010.

U.S. General Accounting Office. Fruits and Vegetables, Enhanced Federal Efforts to Increase Consumption Could Yield Health Benefits for Americans. Washington, D.C.: U.S. General Accounting Office: 2002

Venkatraman JT, Leddy J, Pendergast D: Dietary fats and immune status in athletes: clinical implications. Med Sci Sports Exerc 2000 , 32(7 Suppl):S389-95.

Wolfe RR: Regulation of muscle protein by amino acids. J Nutr 2002.132(10):3219S-24S.

Wurtman, R.J., and J.J. Wurtman. Carbohydrates and depression. Sci Am. 1989. 260(1): 68-75.

Zemel M, Thompson W, Zemel P, Nocton A, Milstead A, Morris K, Campbell P: Dietary calcium and dairy products accelerate weight and fat-loss during energy restriction in obese adults. 2002. Clin Nutri, 75.

Chapter 7

Armstrong, L.E. Heat acclimatization. In: Encyclopedia of Sports Medicine and Science. Internet Society for Sport Science. 1998.

Armstrong LE et al. Table adapted from "The Maintenance of Fluid Balance during Exercise", International Journal of Sports Medicine, 1994; 15(3):122-125.

Armstrong LE, Curtis WC, Hubbard RW, Francesconi RP, Moore R, Askew W. Symptomatic hyponatremia during prolonged exercise in the heat. Med Sci Sports Exerc. 1993;25:543-9.

Ayus JC et al. Hyponatremia, Cerebral Edema, and on cardiogenic Pulmonary Edema in Marathon Runners. Annals of Internal Medicine. 2000;132(9):711-715.

Baker LB, Dougherty KA, Chow M, Kenney WL. Progressive dehydration causes a progressive decline in basketball skill performance. Med Sci Sports Exerc. 2007;39(7):1114–1123.

Burke LM. Nutrition for post-exercise recovery. Aust J Sci Med Sport 1997;29(1):3-10.

Casa D et al. Association Position Statement: Fluid Replacement for Athletes Journal of Athletic Training. Journal of Athletic Training. 2000;35(2): 212-224.

Costill DL et al Muscle Water and Electrolyte Balance During Chronic Exposure and Work in the Heat. 1985; 36.

Coyle, E.F. Fluid and fuel intake during exercise. Journal of Sports Sciences. 2004; 22: 39-55.

Dougherty KA. Two Percent Dehydration Impairs and Six Percent Carbohydrate Drink Improves Boys Basketball Skills. Medicine & Science in Sports & Exercise. 2006;38(9):1650-1658.

Geliebter A. Gastric distension and gastric capacity in relation to food intake in humans, Physiol Behav, 1988; 44:665-8

http://www.sportsdietitians.com.au/www/html/1942-fluids-in-sport.asp Sports Dieticians Australia. Fact Sheet 1, Fluids in Sports. October 25, 2010

Osterberg KL, Horswill CA, and Baker LB. Pregame Urine Specific Gravity and Fluid Intake

by National Basketball Association Players During Competition. Journal of Athletic Training 2009;44(1):53–57.

Shirreffs, S.M., Armstrong, L.E. and Cheuvront, S.N. Fluid and electrolyte needs for preparation and recovery from training and competition. Journal of Sports Sciences. 2004;22, 57-63.

Sawka, M.N., Burke, L.M., Eichner, E.R., Maughan, R.J., Montain, S.J. and Stachen¬field, N.S. American College of Sports Medicine position stand: Exercise and Fluid Replacement. Medicine and Science in Sports and Exercise, 2007;39, 377-390.

Sawka, M N, Wenger CB, Young AJ and Pandolf KB. Physiological responses to exercise in the heat. In: Nutritional Needs in Hot Environments, B.M. Marriott (Ed.). Washington, D.C.: National Academy Press, 1993;55-74.

Sims ST et al. Preexercise sodium loading aids fluid balance and endurance for women exercising in the heat. J Appl Physiol. 2007; 103: 534-541.

Sodium content tomato juice. Accessed at http://www.campbellwellness.com/ product-list.asp?brandCatID=766&brandID=9&productID=2459&cat ID=313 on November 5, 2010.

Volpe, SL, Poule, KA, and Bland EG. Estimation of Prepractice Hydration Status of National

Collegiate Athletic Association Division I Athletes. Journal of Athletic Training 2009;44(6):624–629.

Yeargin SW et al. Thermoregulatory Responses and Hydration Practices in Heat-Acclimatized Adolescents During Preseason High School Football. J Athl Train. 2010; 45(2): 136–146.

The Effect of Different Forms of Fluid Provision on Exercise Performance", International Journal of Sports Medicine. 1993;14:298.

Chapter 8

Gordon, S. Testosterone patch restores libido in postmenopausal women. 2008; Available from: http://health.usnews.com/health-news/family-health/womenshealth/articles/2008/11/05/testosterone-patch-restores-libido-in.html.

Calfee, R. and P. Fadale, Popular ergogenic drugs and supplements in young athletes. Pediatrics, 2006. 117(3): p. e577-89.

Collins, R. Anabolic steroids and the athlete: legal issues. 1999; Available from: www.mesomorphosis.com.

Cussons, A.J., et al., Brown-Séquard revisited: a lesson from history on the placebo effect of androgen treatment. The Med J of Aus, 2002(11-12): p. 678-679.

Peters, J. The man behind the juice: fifty years ago, a doctor brought steroids to America. Slate 2005; Available from: http://www.slate.com/id/2113752/.

Hawley, J.A. and J.O. Holloszy, Exercise: it's the real thing! Nutr Rev, 2009. 67(3): p. 172-8

Hoffman, J.R., et al., Position stand on androgen and human growth hormone use. J Strength Cond Res, 2009. 23(5 Suppl): p. S1-S59.

Liow, R.Y. and S. Tavares, Bilateral rupture of the quadriceps tendon associated with anabolic steroids. Br J Sports Med, 1995. 29(2): p. 77-9.

Eggers, K., NCAA athletes on the juice?, in Portland Tribune. 2005: Portland.

Nussey, S. and S. Whitehead, eds. Endocrinology: An Integrated Approach. 2001, BIOS Scientific Publishers Ltd: Oxford.

Herbst, K.L. and S. Bhasin, Testosterone action on skeletal muscle. Curr Opin Clin Nutr Metab Care, 2004. 7(3): p. 271-7.

Kadi, F., Cellular and molecular mechanisms responsible for the action of testosterone on human skeletal muscle. A basis for illegal performance enhancement. Br J Pharmacol, 2008. 154(3): p. 522-8.

Maravelias, C., et al., Adverse effects of anabolic steroids in athletes. A constant threat. Toxicol Lett, 2005. 158(3): p. 167-75.

Gerber, P.A., et al., The dire consequences of doping. Lancet, 2008. 372(9639): p. 656.

Quaglio, G., et al., Anabolic steroids: dependence and complications of chronic use. Intern Emerg Med, 2009. 4(4): p. 289-96.

Vanberg, P. and D. Atar, Androgenic anabolic steroid abuse and the cardiovascular system. Handb Exp Pharmacol, 2010(195): p. 411-57.

Achar, S., A. Rostamian, and S.M. Narayan, Cardiac and metabolic effects of anabolic androgenic steroid abuse on lipids, blood pressure, left ventricular dimensions, and rhythm. Am J Cardiol, 2010. 106(6): p. 893-901.

Brower, K.J., Anabolic steroid abuse and dependence. Curr Psychiatry Rep, 2002. 4(5): p. 377 87.

Pagonis, T.A., et al., Psychiatric side effects induced by supraphysiological doses of combinations of anabolic steroids correlate to the severity of abuse. Eur Psychiatry, 2006. 21(8): p. 551-62.

Trenton, A.J. and G.W. Currier, Behavioural manifestations of anabolic steroid use. CNS Drugs, 2005. 19(7): p. 571-95.

Midgley, S.J., N. Heather, and J.B. Davies, Levels of aggression among a group of anabolic androgenic steroid users. Med Sci Law, 2001. 41(4): p. 309-14.

Kanayama, G., et al., Treatment of anabolic-androgenic steroid dependence: Emerging evidence and its implications. Drug Alcohol Depend, 2010. 109(1-3): p. 6-13.

Wollina, U., et al., Side-effects of topical androgenic and anabolic substances and steroids. A short review. Acta Dermatovenerol Alp Panonica Adriat, 2007. 16(3): p. 117-22.

Horn, S., P. Gregory, and K.M. Guskiewicz, Self-reported anabolic-androgenic steroids use and musculoskeletal injuries: findings from the center for the study of retired athletes health survey of retired NFL players. Am J Phys Med Rehabil, 2009. 88(3): p. 192-200.

Schwingel, P.A., et al., Anabolic-androgenic steroids: a possible new risk factor of toxicant associated fatty liver disease. Liver Int, 2010.

Hama, H., T. Yamamuro, and T. Takeda, Experimental studies on connective tissue of the capsular ligament. Influences of aging and sex hormones. Acta Orthop Scand, 1976. 47(5): p. 473-9.

Rich, J.D., et al., Abscess related to anabolic-androgenic steroid injection. Med Sci Sports Exerc, 1999. 31(2): p. 207-9.

Fainaru-Wada, M. Former NFL lineman pleads guilty to lying to feds. 2008; Available from: http://sports.espn.go.com/nfl/news/story?id=3202950.

Schrotenboer, B., A detailed history, in San Deigo Tribune. 2008.

Patrick, D. DEA nets largest steroid bust. USA Today 2007; Available from: http://www.usatoday.com/sports/olympics/2007-09-24-DEA-steroid-bust_N.htm. (2005) DEA leads largest steroid bust in history.

Kreider, R.B., et al., ISSN exercise & sport nutrition review: research & recommendations. J Int Soc Sports Nutr, 2010. 7: p. 7.

Dalbo, V.J., et al., Putting to rest the myth of creatine supplementation leading to muscle cramps and dehydration. Br J Sports Med, 2008. 42(7): p. 567-73.

Dohrmann, G. Is this Dr. Evil? SI Vault 2006; Available from: http://sportsillustrated.cnn.com/vault/article/magazine/MAG1104278/2/index.htm.

Willoughby, D.S., et al., Eight weeks of aromatase inhibition using the nutritional supplement Novedex XT: effects in young, eugonadal men. Int J Sport Nutr Exerc Metab, 2007. 17(1): p. 92 108.

Rohle, D., et al., Effects of eight weeks of an alleged aromatase inhibiting nutritional supplement 6-OXO (androst-4-ene-3,6,17-trione) on serum hormone profiles and clinical safety markers in resistance-trained, eugonadal males. J Int Soc Sports Nutr, 2007. 4: p. 13.

Wingert, N., H. Tavakoli, and E. Yoder, Acute hepatitis and personality change in a 31-year-old man taking prohormone supplement SUS500. Psychosomatics, 2010. 51(4): p. 340-4.

Kafrouni, M.I., R.A. Anders, and S. Verma, Hepatotoxicity associated with dietary supplements containing anabolic steroids. Clin Gastroenterol Hepatol, 2007. 5(7): p. 809-12.

Krishnan, P.V., Z.Z. Feng, and S.C. Gordon, Prolonged intrahepatic cholestasis and renal failure secondary to anabolic androgenic steroid-enriched dietary supplements. J Clin Gastroenterol, 2009. 43(7): p. 672-5.

Burke, L.M. (2000) Positive Drug Tests from Supplements Sportsicence 4.

Dalbo, V.J., et al., Acute effects of ingesting a commercial thermogenic drink on changes in energy expenditure and markers of lipolysis. J Int Soc Sports Nutr, 2008. 5: p. 6.

Haller, C.A. and N.L. Benowitz, Adverse cardiovascular and central nervous system events associated with dietary supplements containing ephedra alkaloids. N Engl J Med, 2000. 343(25): p. 1833-8.

Holmes, R.O., Jr. and J. Tavee, Vasospasm and stroke attributable to ephedra-free xenadrine: case report. Mil Med, 2008. 173(7): p. 708-10.

Bouchard, N.C., et al., Ischemic stroke associated with use of an ephedra-free dietary supplement containing synephrine. Mayo Clin Proc, 2005. 80(4): p. 541-5.

Thomas, J.E., et al., STEMI in a 24-year-old man after use of a synephrine-containing dietary supplement: a case report and review of the literature. Tex Heart Inst J, 2009. 36(6): p. 586-90.

Stephensen, T.A. and R. Sarlay, Jr., Ventricular fibrillation associated with use of synephrine containing dietary supplement. Mil Med, 2009. 174(12): p. 1313-9.

Hapke, H.J. and W. Strathmann, [Pharmacological effects of hordenine]. Dtsch Tierarztl Wochenschr, 1995. 102(6): p. 228-32.

Lanni, A., et al., 3,5-diiodo-L-thyronine powerfully reduces adiposity in rats by increasing the burning of fats. FASEB J, 2005. 19(11): p. 1552-4.

Grasselli, E., et al., Effects of 3,5-diiodo-L-thyronine administration on the liver of high fat diet fed rats. Exp Biol Med (Maywood), 2008. 233(5): p. 549-57.

Sharma, B., et al., Effects of guggulsterone isolated from Commiphora mukul in high fat diet induced diabetic rats. Food Chem Toxicol, 2009. 47(10): p. 2631-9.

Warning on Hydroxycut Products. 2009; Available from: FDA U.S. Food and Drug

Administration. http://www.fda.gov/ForConsumers/ConsumerUpdates/ucm152152.htm.

Grivetti, L.E. and E.A. Applegate, From Olympia to Atlanta: a cultural-historical perspective on diet and athletic training. J Nutr, 1997. 127(5 Suppl): p. 860S-868S.

Chapter 9

Arthur, M., & Bailey B. (1998). Complete conditioning for football. Champaign, Illinois: Human Kinetics Publishers, Inc.

Bompa, T. (2001). Periodizing training for peak performance. In B. Foran (Ed.), High Performance Sports Conditioning. (pp. 267-282). Champaign, Illinois: Human Kinetics Publishers, Inc.

Boyle, M. (2010). Advances in functional training. Aptos, California: On Target Publications.

Boyle, M. (2004). Functional training for sports. Champaign, Illinois: Human Kinetics Publishers, Inc.

Clark, M., & Russell, A. (2007). Postural considerations. Calabasas, California: National Academy of Sports Medicine.

Clark, M., & Russell, A. (2007). Integrated program design. Calabasas, California: National Academy of Sports Medicine.

Coker, C. (2009). Motor learning & control. Scottsdale, Arizona: Holcomb Hathaway, Publishers, Inc.

Gleim, G. W., & McHugh, M. P. (1997). Flexibility and its effects on sports injury and performance. Sports Med 24(5), 289-299.

Issurin, V. (2008). Block periodization: breakthrough in sport training. Michigan: Ultimate Athlete Concepts.

Kenn, J. (2002). Strength training playbook for coaches. USA.

Kraemer, W., & Gomez, A. (2001). Establishing a Solid Fitness Base. In B. Foran (Ed.), High Performance Sports Conditioning. (pp. 3-17). Champaign, Illinois: Human Kinetics Publishers, Inc.

Kraemer, W. J., & Fleck , S. J. (2005). Strength training for young athletes (2nd ed.). Champaign, Illinois: Human Kinetics Publishers, Inc.

Matveyev, L. (1997). Fundamentals of sport training. Moscow: Progress Publishers.

Baechle, T. R., & Earle, R. W. (2008) Essentials of strength training and conditioning (3rd ed.). National Strength and Conditioning Association. Champaign, Illinois: Human Kinetics Publishers, Inc.

Plisk, S. S. (2001). Muscular strength and stamina. In B. Foran (Ed.), High

Performance Sports Conditioning. (pp. 63-82). Champaign, Illinois: Human Kinetics Publishers, Inc.

Thrash, K., Kelly, B. (1987). Flexibility and strength training. Journal of Applied Sports Science Research 1(4), 74-75.

Vermeil, A., Helland, E., & Gattone, M. (1999). Vermeil's sports and fitness training system for enhancing athletic performance. Vermeil's Sports and Fitness.

Viru, A. (1995). Adaptation in sports training. Boca Raton, Florida: CRC Press

Zatsiorsky, V. M. (1995). Science and practice of strength training. Champaign, Illinois: Human Kinetics Publishers, Inc.

Yessis, M. (2006). Build a better athlete. Terre Haute, Indiana: Equilibrium Books

Chapter 10

Arthur, M., & Bailey B. (1998). Complete conditioning for football. Champaign, Illinois: Human Kinetics Publishers, Inc.

Baechle, T. R., & Earle, R. W. (2008) Essentials of strength training and conditioning (3rd ed.). National Strength and Conditioning Association. Champaign, Illinois: Human Kinetics Publishers, Inc.

Berg, K. (1982). Anaerobic conditioning: training the three energy systems. National Strength Coaches Association Journal 4(1), 48-50.

Boyle, M. (2010). Advances in functional training. Aptos, California: On Target Publications.

Boyle, M. (2004). Functional training for sports. Champaign, Illinois: Human Kinetics Publishers, Inc.

Etcheberry, P. (1985). College football conditioning at the University of Wisconson. National Strength Coaches Association Journal. 4(4), 26-33.

Francis, C. (2008). Key concepts 2008 elite edition. Charlie Francis.com.

Gaesser, G. A., & Wilson, L. A. (1988). Effects of continuous and interval training on the parameters of the power-endurance time relationship for high-intensity exercise. International Journal of Sports Medicine. 9(6), 417-421.

Karp, J. (2010). Strength training for distance running: a scientific perspective. Strength & Conditioning Journal. 32(3), 83-86.

Kenn, J. (2002). Strength training playbook for coaches. USA.

Kraemer, W., & Gomez, A. (2001). Establishing a Solid Fitness Base. In B. Foran (Ed.), High Performance Sports Conditioning. (pp. 3-17). Champaign, Illinois: Human Kinetics Publishers, Inc.

Lapoff, D. (2002). Use of the exhaustive performance curve to prescribe anaerobic intervals: part 1. Strength & Conditioning Journal. 24(2), 34-35.

Lapoff, D. (2002). Use of the exhaustive performance curve to prescribe anaerobic intervals: part 2. Strength & Conditioning Journal. 24(3), 37-39.

Palmer, M. S., & Potteiger, J. A. (1996). Understanding the lactate threshold. Strength & Conditioning. 18(1), 42-25.

Plisk, S. S. (2001). Muscular strength and stamina. In B. Foran (Ed.), High Performance Sports Conditioning. (pp. 63-82). Champaign, Illinois: Human Kinetics Publishers, Inc.

Plisk, S. S. (1991). Anaerobic metabolic conditioning: a brief review of theory, strategy and practical application. Journal of Applied Sport Science Research. 5(1), 22-34.

Schoenfeld, B., & Dawes, J. (2009). High-intensity interval training: applications for general fitness training. Strength & Conditioning Journal. 31(6), 44-46.

Taylor, J. (2004). A tactical metabolic training model for collegiate basketball. Strength & Conditioning Journal. 26(5), 22-29.

Vermeil, A., Helland, E., & Gattone, M. (1999). Vermeil's sports and fitness training system for enhancing athletic performance. Vermeil's Sports and Fitness.

Viru, A. (1995). Adaptation in sports training. Boca Raton, Florida: CRC Press

Watts, J. H. (1996). Sport specific conditioning for anaerobic athletes. Strength & Conditioning. 18(4), 33-36.